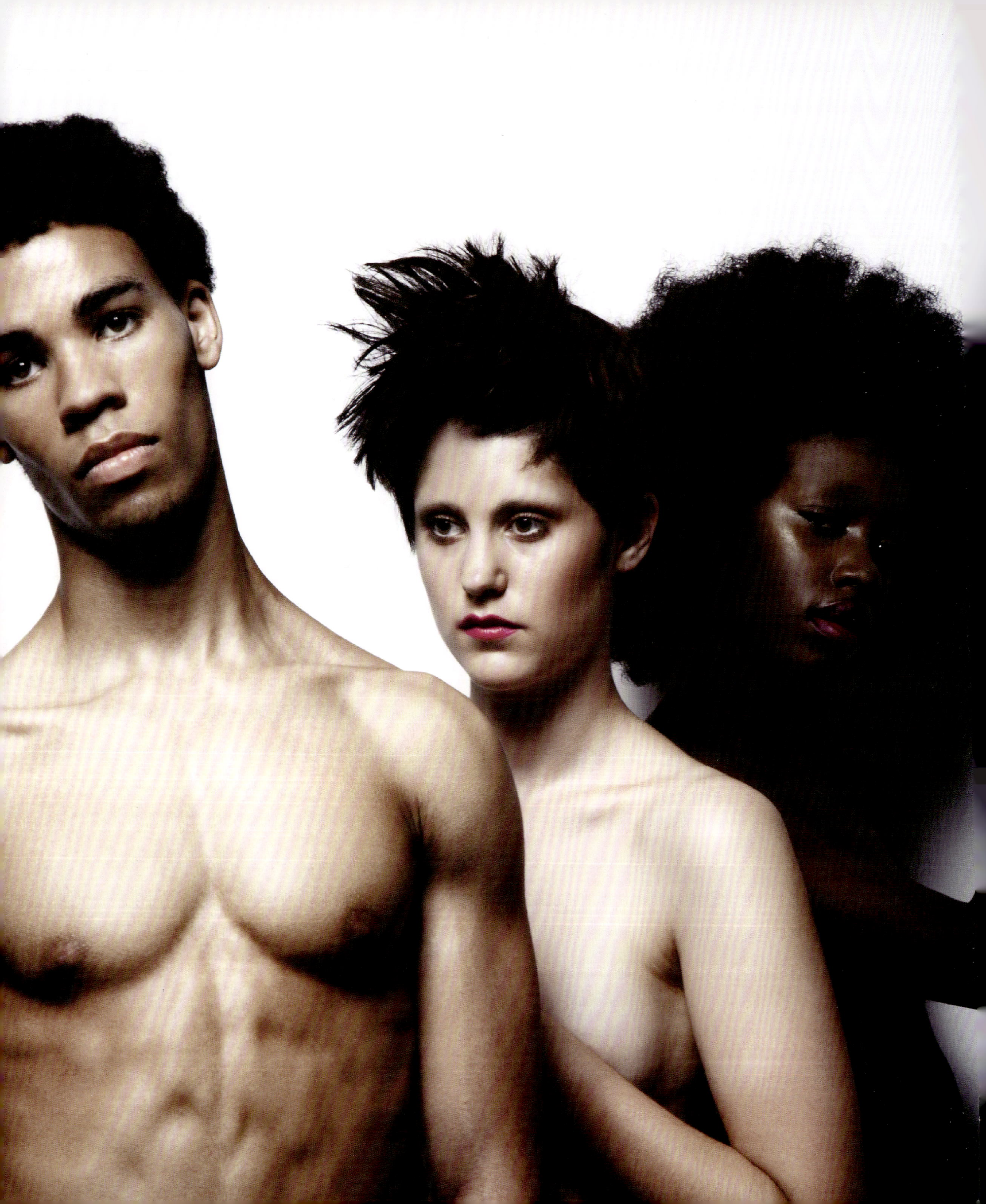

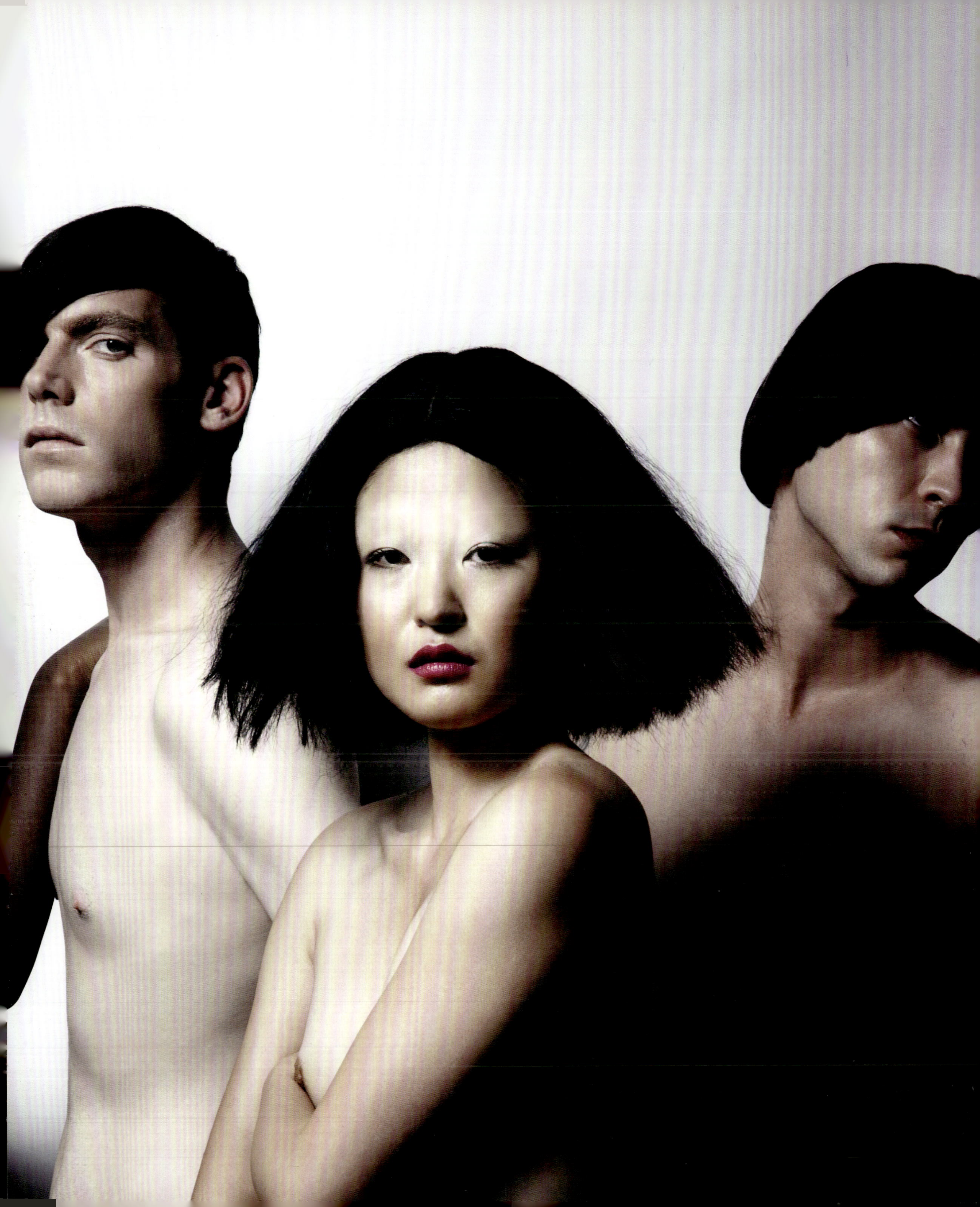

Acknowledgments

Hair by Roy Hayward

Thank you to everyone involved in technique. Nigel d' Auvergne, Mike Bliss, Natasha Bloom, James Brown, Pete Brown, Anita Brulee, Cheryl Corea, Britt Cormack, Valentina Creti, Christabel Draffin, Lucy Flower, Jonathan Haynes, Maxine Henshilwood, Margo Holder, Lena Hrncarova, Greg Jakobek, Tony James, Junichi Kikuchi, Valerie Klym, Paul Krokos, Anne Lueck, Ashley Rae, Gail Rhodes, Mark Rowley, Valentina Salaris, Matthew Salisbury, Naomi Selig, Jenny Svantesson, Kristina Theodoris, Richard Turgoose and a very special thank you to all the models.

British Library Cataloguing-in-Publication Data. A catalogue record of this book is available from the British Library.

ISBN 978-0-9560323-0-0

First published in the United Kingdom in 2008 by Hardway
Design by Warsaw. Printed by B.A.S

For seminar and course bookings or further information contact:
www.royhayward.com

technique

a complete course in modern hairdressing for men and women

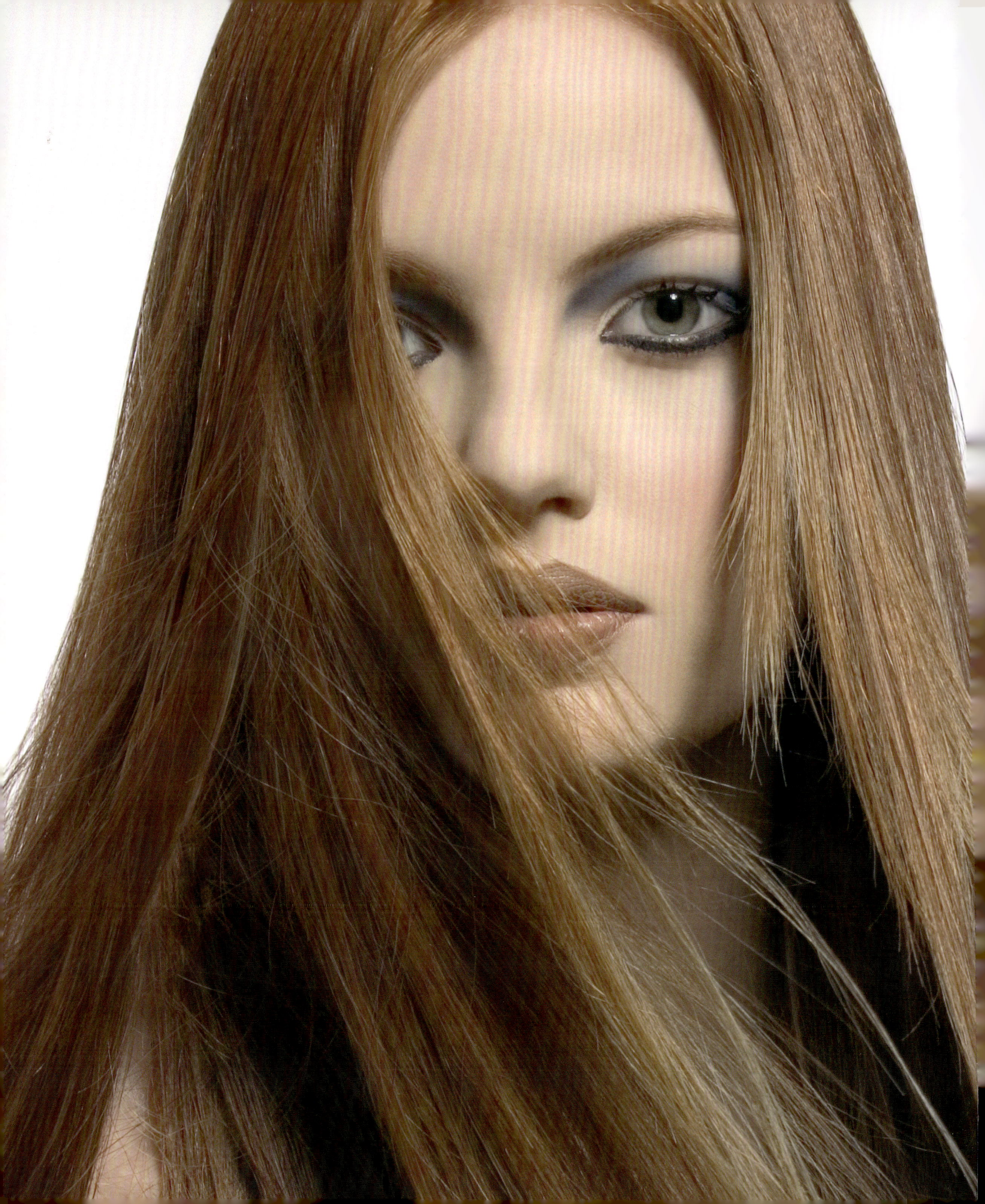

Contents

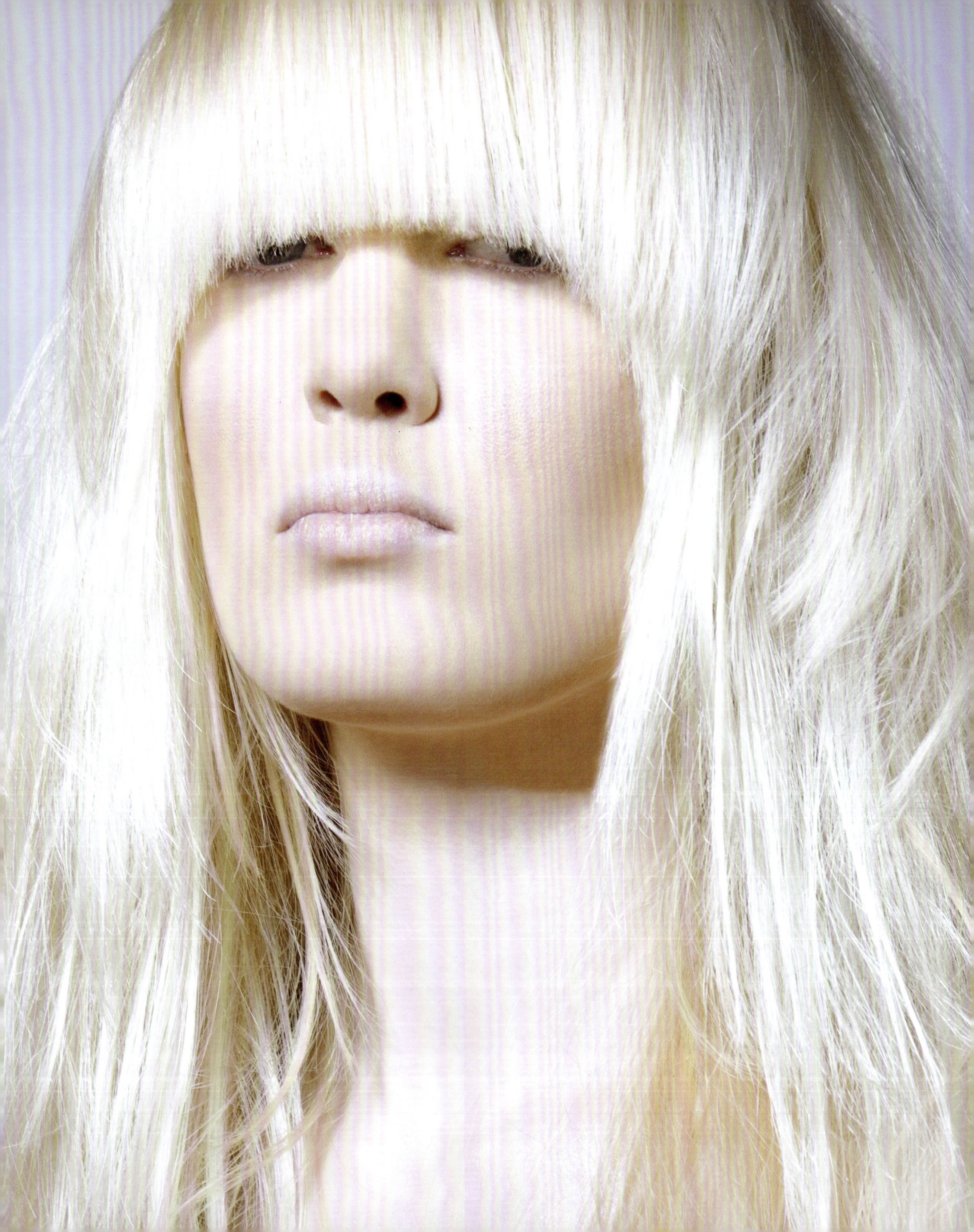

Introducing Technique

Here you will find an educational programme which establishes the foundations of modern hairdressing for today's hairdresser. The main aim of the book is to demonstrate uncomplicated techniques and strong ideas. Each section of the book has been carefully designed to help hairdressers acquire a progressive approach and achieve the highest standards in their work.

The book will reinforce and refine any previously learnt knowledge to give you a technical and creative edge. A thorough mastery of the techniques in this book will give you the foundations on which all advanced, commercial and fashion techniques are based.

This is a complete hairdressing programme that includes easy-to-follow step-by-step techniques in all aspects of hairdressing. By using this book as a guide, you will gradually increase your confidence and expertise. The book covers shapes, textures, colour, methods and many more areas in hairdressing and will set you apart as you move towards becoming a professional hairdresser.

Training and education are of paramount importance in hairdressing, as they represent an investment in the service offered to the client. As you will come to see, the sharing of knowledge and ideas takes place at all levels in the industry, and is an essential way of keeping up with developments. For those considering a career in hairdressing, you should ideally have a certain degree of artistic flair. You'll need good hand and eye coordination and dexterity. Your personality should be sparkling, strong and interesting. You'll need to have a good level of physical stamina. The basic rules of anatomy, biology, chemistry and psychology will be part of your learning.

You will be working in a creative atmosphere and should have the ability to be an excellent communicator, as you'll be working with people from every age group and background. In addition you'll need to be a good listener and be diplomatic and sympathetic towards clients and colleagues.

In an ever-changing, fast moving and exciting industry the opportunities are endless for a highly rewarding career.

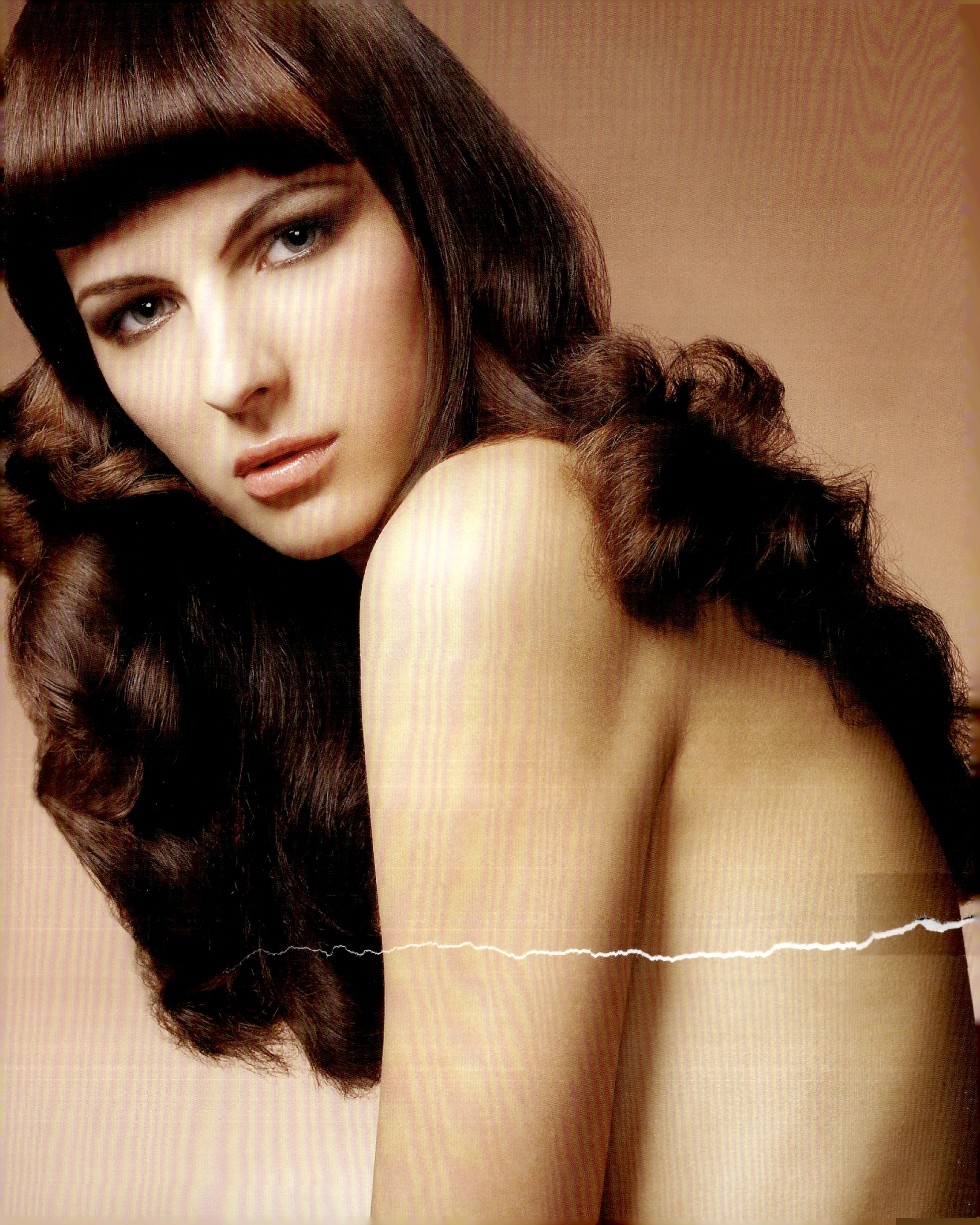

Hairdressing — A Career Guide

The world of hairdressing offers many choices; the following examples explain where a career in hairdressing may take you.

The Salon

A hairdresser generally works from the salon, and the training period usually lasts between two and three years. A hairdresser can choose to cover all aspects of hairdressing, providing the client with cutting, styling and technical services. Some hairdressers specialise in cutting and styling only and work as salon stylists, and some specialise in technical services and work as salon technicians.

Once you are a qualified stylist you can progress to becoming a style or artistic director, perhaps an educational director or even a salon manager. Salons can vary in size, from the many recognisable high street chains to the well-established smaller independent salons. In a fast moving, exciting and creative industry being a salon-based hairdresser can be highly rewarding and a very satisfying career.

Film, Television and Theatre

You will need some experience and a qualification in wig-making and possibly make-up, plus some practical experience with theatrical companies. Film, television and theatre companies have thousands of applications each year for very few places, so there are very limited openings in these areas. Television, for instance, is a highly competitive field. You should have good hair and make-up skills as well as being an excellent communicator. You will need to be prepared to work all sorts of hours as 'call time' can mean a very early start, especially when working on a film or television production.

If you decide to pursue a hairdressing career in film or television you may spend long periods of time away on location filming. In theatre, the company and production may spend weeks or months on tour so, again, you'll be spending time away from home. Hairdressers naturally possess good people skills, something needed within this particular branch of the industry, especially when you come into contact with celebrities and high profile actors.

Working for a Manufacturer

Large manufacturers of hairdressing products and equipment usually employ hairdressers in the following areas.

Sales Representatives sell products to hairdressers. Sales reps are often based in their own designated area within the country and will be responsible for area sales and coordination.

Technical Representatives give technical advice and support on products and services. You may visit salons to demonstrate new or existing products, or you may give technical support and advice to salons over the phone from your head office or branch.

Educators demonstrate the use of hairdressing products, services and techniques, often working from salons, training centres, colleges or within the manufacturer's own schools. As an educator you may need a teaching qualification or an educational diploma from the company that you wish to represent.

Session Hairdressing

A session hairdresser creates hairstyles for national and international fashion shows, advertising campaigns, fashion magazine editorial shoots, catalogues, music videos, TV and film. A session hairdresser is usually represented by an agency which specialises in this field of work. You will need a portfolio of your work. This should include a general selection of the quality photographic work you have created. High fashion and commercial work will often be included in your portfolio. Mostly you will be working for fashion magazines, and newspapers, shooting editorial work. Advertising campaigns for high profile companies can be very lucrative and prestigious. You may also work on top models' hair at fashion shows at fashion weeks in London, Paris, Milan and New York.

Before becoming a session stylist you will need to have gained a lot of experience in all aspects of hairdressing. This area is very competitive and success is determined by your skills and ability. When you start out you'll often find yourself working for nothing, assisting other session hairdressers as a means of demonstrating your abilities. This is very common at the early stages of session work and allows you to build up your book, which will prepare you for finding an agent. Session hairdressing is hard work and requires lots of stamina. You will come into contact with many creative people in the fashion industry such as other industry professionals like photographers, models, fashion stylists, make-up artists, magazine editors, fashion designers and artistic directors.

Session hairdressers can work in areas where conditions are hectic, and where the location will depend on where the session is going to be. They often work unsupervised but may supervise others such as assistants or a team of people. Maturity and self-confidence is needed in this area of hairdressing as well as the ability to work under pressure and to meet deadlines. You should have good time management skills and creative flair, design and colour sense.

Teaching

Once you gain in salon experience as a stylist you could progress to teaching in a college, training centre or salon academy. To assess students you must obtain your A1 award. To be able to teach you'll need a qualification such as City and Guilds 7407, which is a widely recognised teaching qualification. A tutor of hairdressing will usually teach on a National Vocational Qualification programme in a college: the tutor is responsible for monitoring and ensuring the progress of students. The NVQ is very basic and there is often a good deal of paperwork involved in this area of teaching. The NVQ programme consists of levels one, two and three. Alternatively you may want to teach on a programme or course which has been developed to a salon or academy's own standards. A thorough knowledge of the particular programme will be needed. Be prepared to go through retraining to reach the exacting level required.

Trichology

Hairdressers often refer clients with hair and scalp disorders to a trichologist. A trichologist is a hair and scalp specialist who deals with various problems such as hair loss, problematic scalp, alopecia, etc. It takes several years to qualify with the Institute of Trichologists. Once qualified, you could find work in either a hair clinic or a hairdressing salon.

It is often said that you never stop learning in hairdressing. You have chosen one of the most stimulating, exciting and demanding careers around.

A career in hairdressing can progress in many different directions: you could become a famous celebrity hairdresser with your own product range, or you may dream of owning your own salon one day or perhaps working in the film or television world. There are many possibilities.

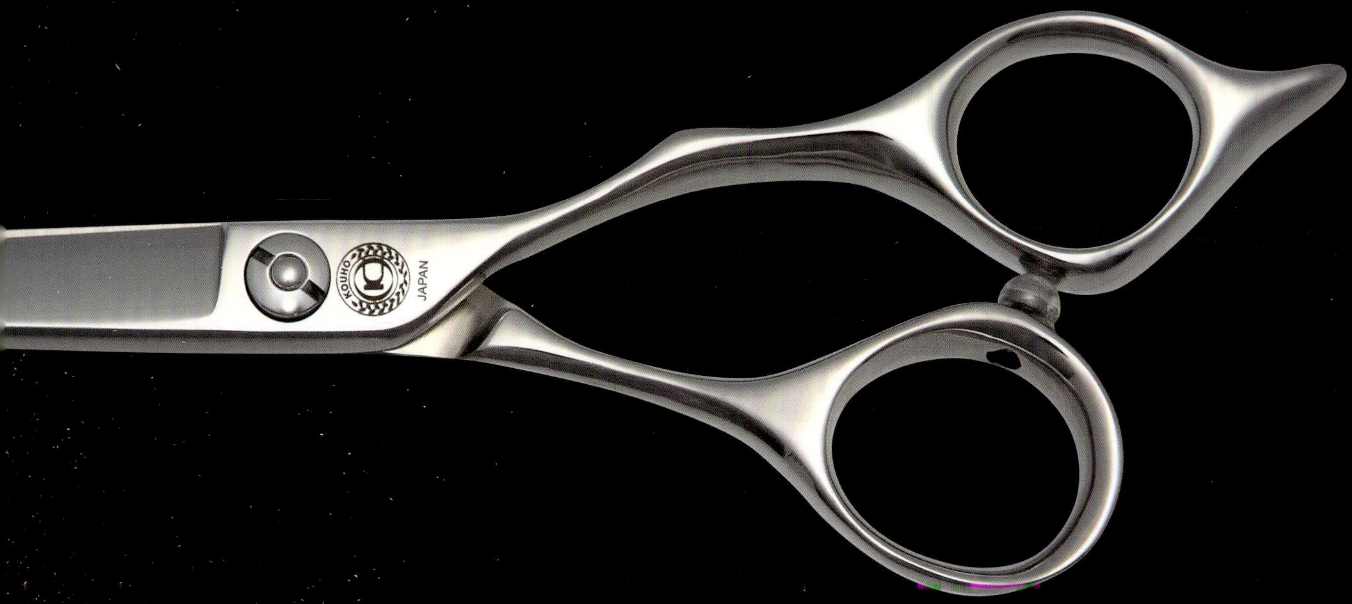
KOUHO
JAPAN

Equipment

In hairdressing it is especially important that you work with tools of a high quality to carry out the services that the client requires. Always invest in good quality equipment.

Scissors

Clients visit the salon more frequently for a haircut than for any other service, so it is worth investing first in good quality scissors. Scissors are made from tempered or cobalt steel and are available in various sizes, measuring from 10cm to 18cm from the tip of the blade to the handles. Many hairdressers prefer to use short scissors for precision cutting: longer scissors are useful for other techniques such as texturising.

Always take good care of your scissors and never use them for cutting anything other than hair, or they will quickly become blunt. Keep the blades dry after each haircut by wiping them with cotton wool and surgical spirit (this will also disinfect them).

Lightly oil the blades and the pivot screw if they start to feel stiff and awkward to use.

Try not to drop your scissors as the blades may become damaged and the pivot screw (which balances the scissors) could work loose.

Keep your scissors in their original protective case for safety and to prevent them from becoming damaged.

If they need mending or sharpening, always send them to a professional hairdressing scissor company. Choose your scissors carefully: they must feel comfortable to work with. Try before you buy: hold scissors to see how they feel.

You can always spot professional hairdressers by the way they pick up and hold a pair of scissors, using the thumb and third finger. They do this to achieve maximum control during cutting.

Before starting a haircut always adjust the height of the chair or bend from your knees, keeping your back straight. Body position is very important for the hairdresser during cutting. A cutting stool is an excellent idea as it allows you to work at the correct height and can be moved around the client.

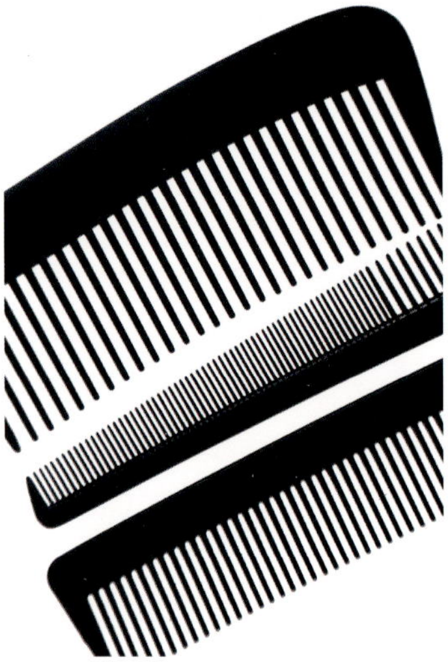

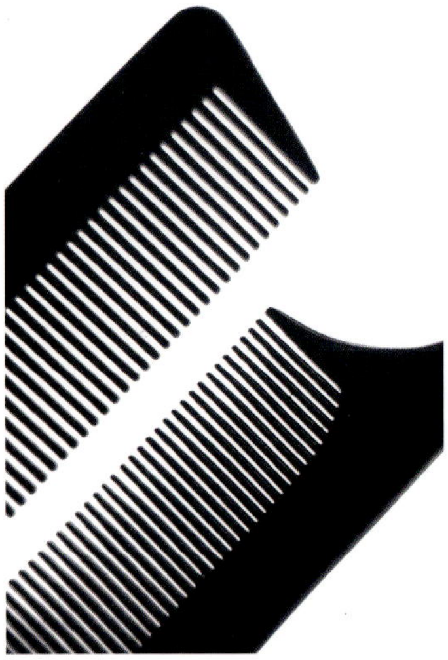

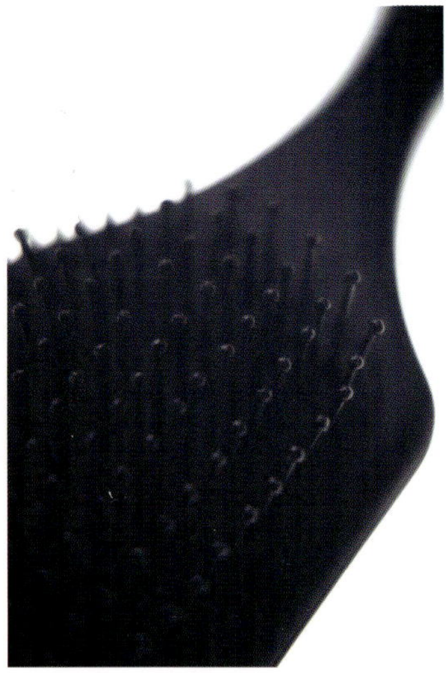

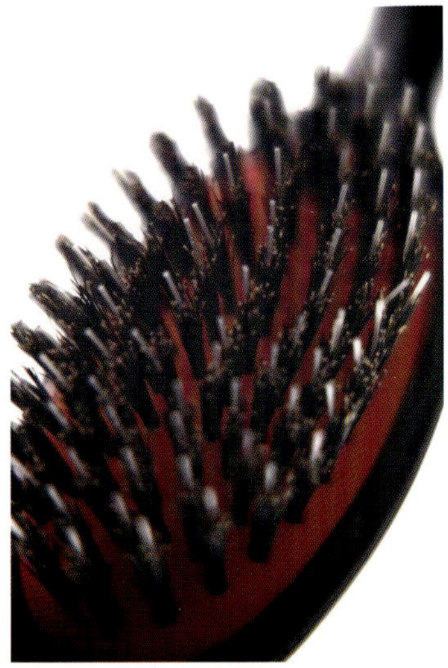

Combs

Good quality cutting combs are made from vulcanised rubber with tapered teeth. This type of comb is particularly useful when employing scissor-over-comb techniques, and will give you great results. Avoid metal and plastic combs as they tend to rip and split hair.

Combs made of vulcanised rubber are much more flexible and do not harm the hair or scalp in any way; and they are easily cleaned, guarding against germs and cross-infection. All combs found in your kit should be made from vulcanised rubber including tail combs, pin tail combs, barbering combs, and wide-tooth combs.

Brushes

A variety of brushes are useful for achieving various effects and finishes, especially for blow drying and styling. Good quality brushes are made from high performance materials and are available in various sizes and bristle types. Always work with the correct brush to achieve the desired effect and finish.

Paddle brushes are excellent for de-tangling and preparing hair, and come in various sizes. The ball end bristles are supported on a cushioned rubber base which helps eliminate static electricity.

Natural bristle brushes are often made from wild boar bristle. The bristle or quill is supported on an air-cushioned rubber base. This type of brush is often favoured by session stylists as it's a perfect tool for smoothing and dressing out hair.

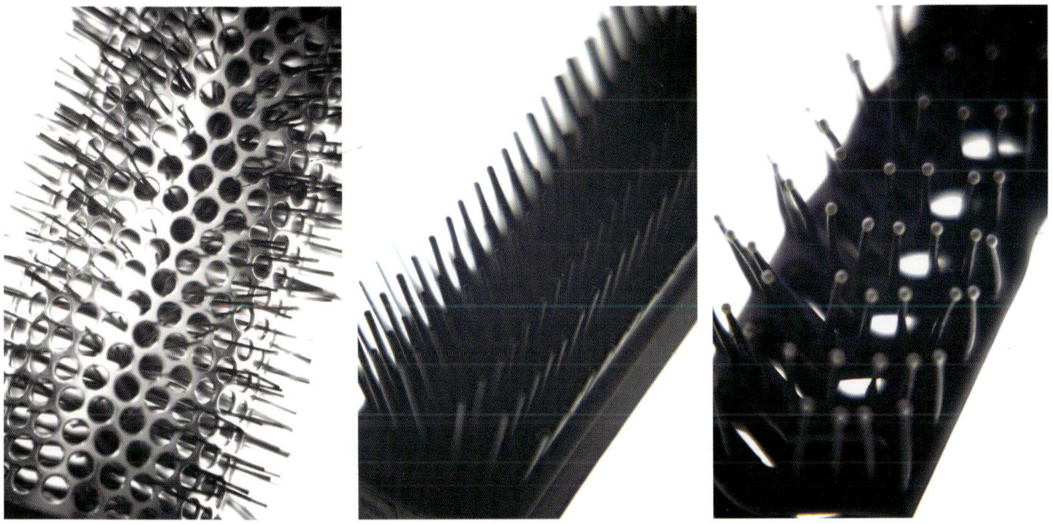

Radial ceramic brushes are available in a variety of sizes with a ceramic coated barrel and either natural or nylon bristle; these brushes are excellent for smoothing and straightening hair. A radial brush will also give movement, root lift, volume and curl to your client's hair. A radial ceramic provides good heat retention as the brush is designed to conduct heat evenly from the dryer, creating a smooth glossy finish.

Styling brushes are available in various sizes and are usually made from an anti-static rubber base with nylon bristles which have rounded ends. This particular brush is suitable for use on most types and length of hair. The base is easily removable, making the brush very easy to clean for maintaining hygiene.

Vent brushes are made with ball end bristles and are designed to allow the flow of air from the hairdryer to pass directly through a series of chevron vents at the base of the brush. Vent brushes are also excellent at de-tangling without pulling or damaging hair. They are particularly useful when blow drying curly hair. The vent brush is more commonly used for men's hairstyling as less volume in the finish is usually required in men's hairstyling.

In styling and finishing hair you will be using a variety of brushes. Your choice of brush will be influenced by the particular finish required. The size of brush also depends on the length of hair you will be working on. Make sure you feel comfortable when handling your brushes.

Neck brushes are used to eliminate hair from your client's face and neck.

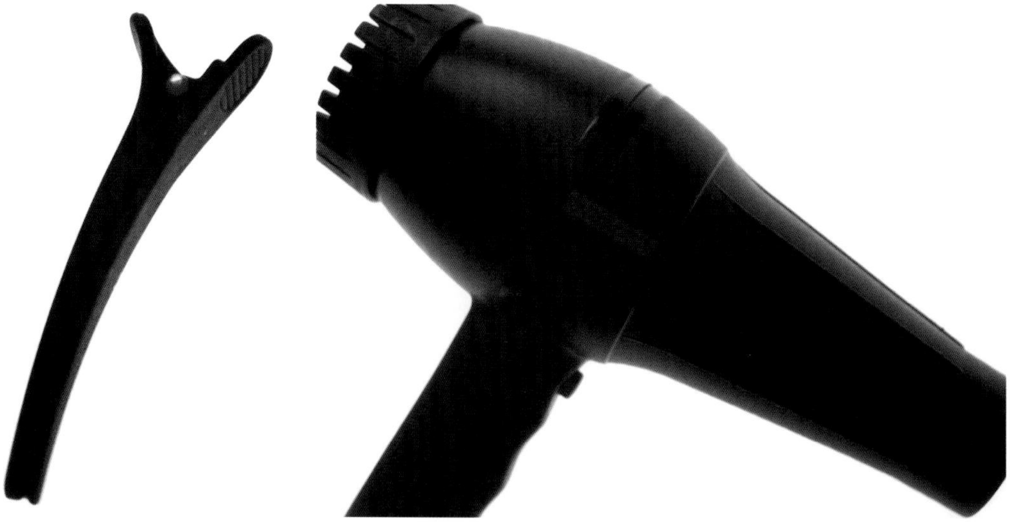

Section Clips

These are an essential tool for holding hair away in your section or parting. They are available in metal or plastic and are used for virtually every service in hairdressing.

Hairdryers

They should be strong, powerful and of good quality. Hand-held hairdryers are essential pieces of equipment. Professional hairdryers are designed to be used in the salon continuously and need to be lightweight with adjustable speeds and temperatures.

The key attachments used for the hairdryer are a nozzle and a diffuser. Nozzles concentrate the flow of air from the hairdryer and are often used in blow drying – they help create a smooth finish on hair. Using a diffuser will speed up the process of drying hair off naturally without disturbing the hair.

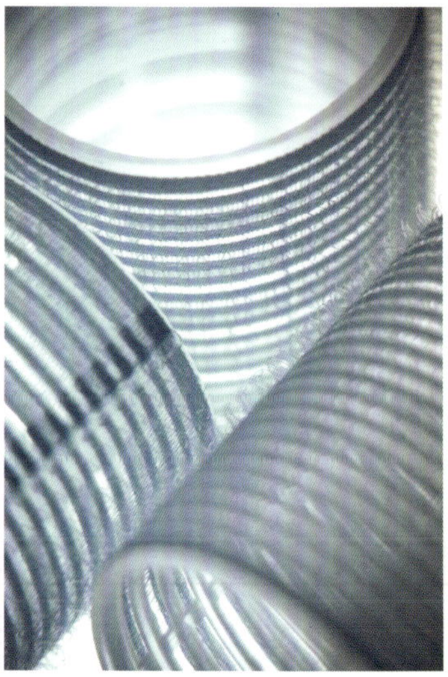

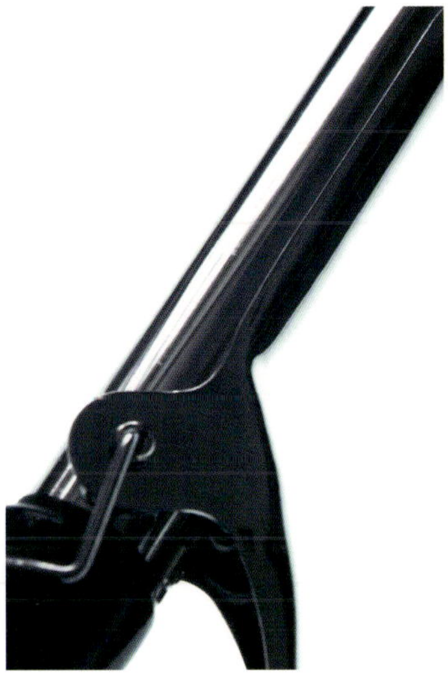

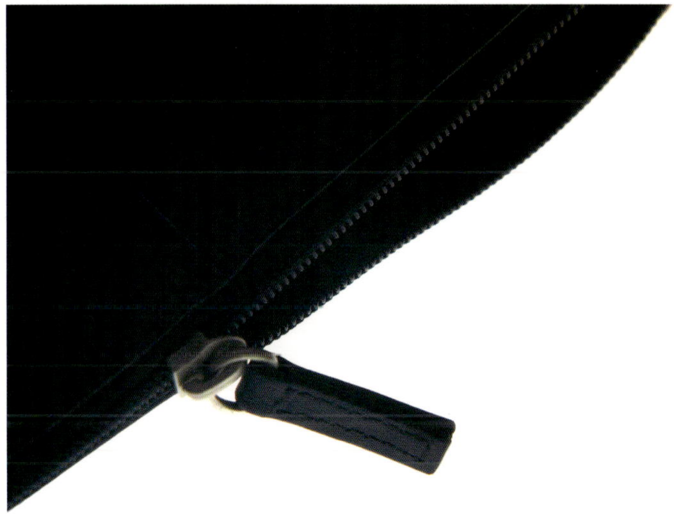

Rollers

Self-grip or Velcro rollers are usually used on dry hair during blow drying – self-grip rollers can be used without pins as they attach easily to hair. Plastic rollers are used for wet setting; this method of setting involves drying under a hood dryer. A hair net should be used before placing a client under a dryer.

Heated rollers are used on dry hair. Rollers for setting hair come in a variety of sizes and are secured and held in place with pins and grips. The type or size of roller used will depend on the effect you want to achieve.

Curling Tongs

Thick-barrelled tongs create soft movement while a smaller barrel will give a tighter more defined curl. Ceramic technology will provide even distribution of heat along the barrel, giving longer-lasting results. Remember tongs remain hot for some time after they are switched off. They are available in various sizes.

A Kit Holder

These will keep your equipment tidy and together; some holders have compartments which your equipment can be slotted into.

Keep all your equipment clean and sterile and ensure that you practise good health and safety procedures. Pay particular attention to combs, scissors and brushes. Your equipment should be cleaned and sterilised immediately after use.

Vocabulary

Partings and Sections

1 **Perimeter**: the outer edge of the haircut. This can also be referred to as a guide or baseline.

2 **Diagonal back section**: a diagonal line which, taken on an angle, works backwards away from the face.

3 **Diagonal forward section**: a diagonal line which, taken on an angle, works forward towards the front of the face.

4 **Halo section**: a circular section which travels back around the head, usually 3cm in from the hairline.

5 **Horizontal section**: parallel to the horizon.

6 **Horseshoe section**: from each recession area on the temple, running through the occipital bone.

7 **Profile line**: a central division from centre forehead to centre nape.

8 **Radial section**: from the top of the crown to the area behind each ear on both sides of the head.

9 **Vertical section**: perpendicular to the horizon.

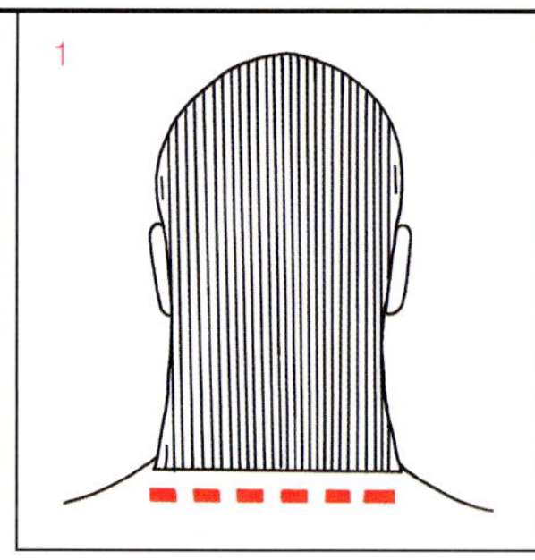

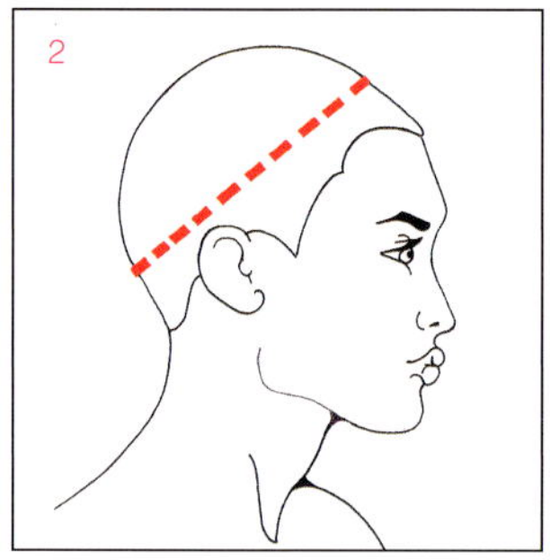

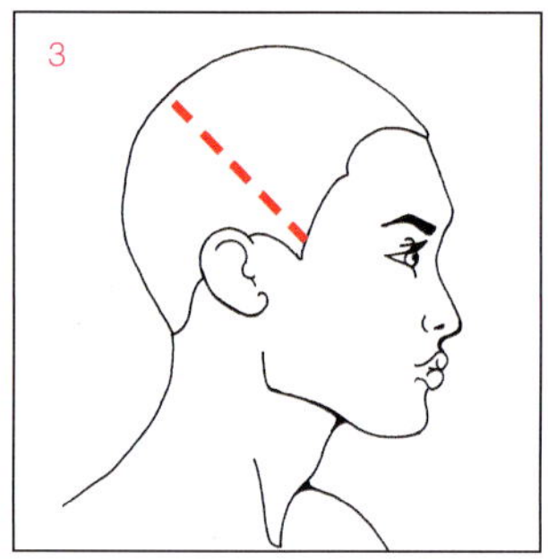

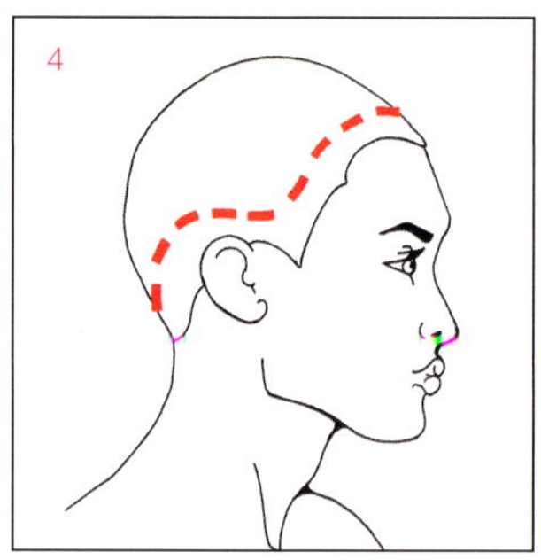

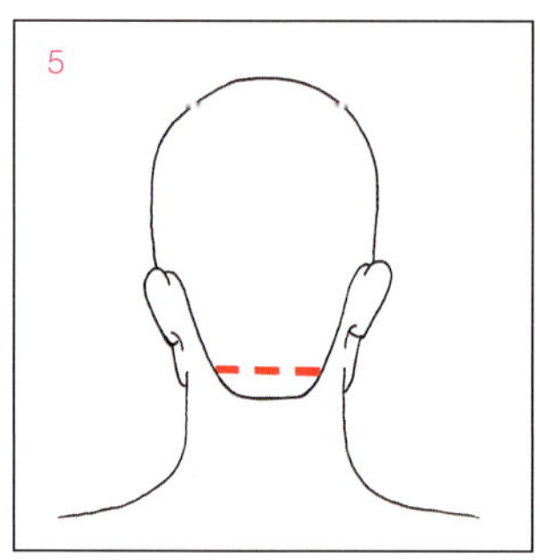

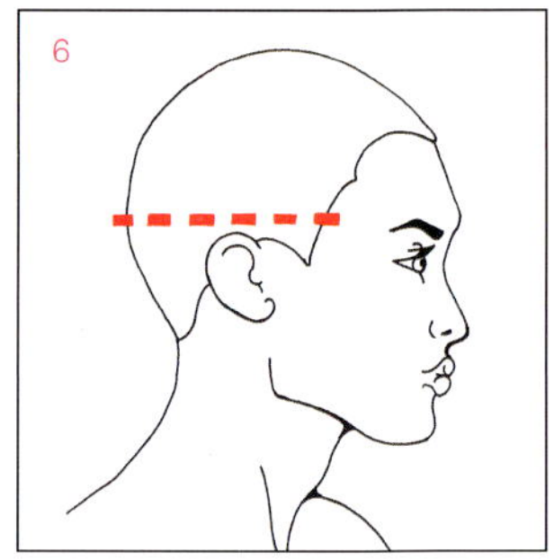

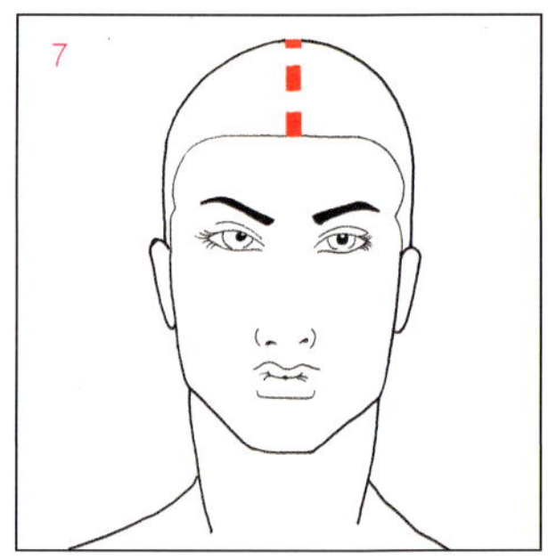

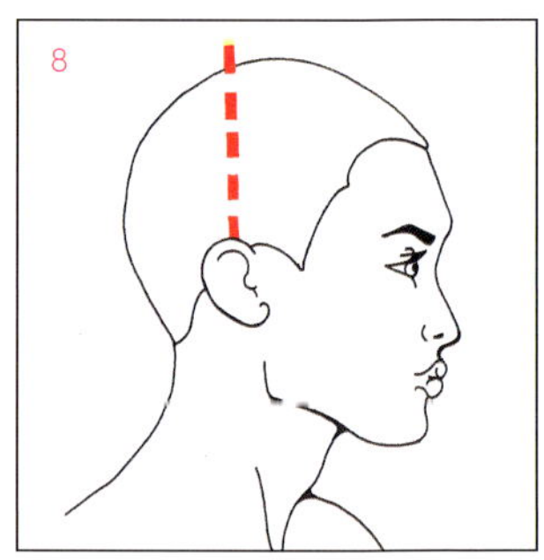

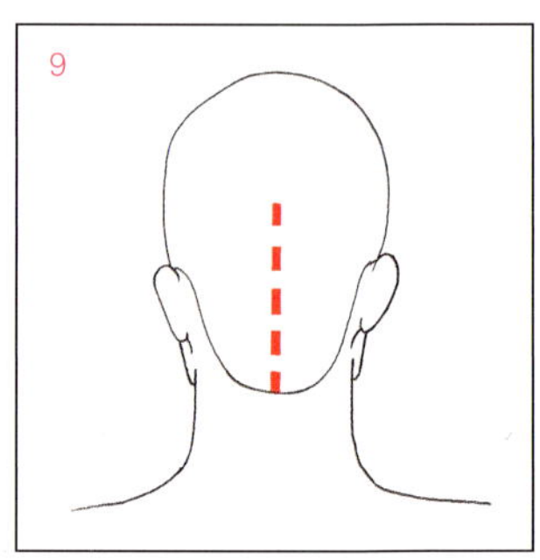

References to the Head

1 **Apex**: where the top of the ear joins the head.

2 **Centre forehead**: from the bridge of the nose, travel up towards the front hairline.

3 **Crown**: usually the highest point and centre of the top of the head. The circular natural growth pattern will be found here.

4 **Growth pattern**: direction of hair growth.

5 **Hairline**: the point at which the growth of hair starts.

6 **Nape area**: the point beneath the hairline at the back of the head, where the neck joins the head.

7 **Occipital bone**: prominent bone at the back of the head – usually protrudes more on men than on women.

8 **Profile**: the side view of the head.

9 **Recession area**: the area of the hairline which is curved – the point between the forehead and the temple area.

10 **Temple area** the area on both sides of the head, above the cheek bones and below the front hairline.

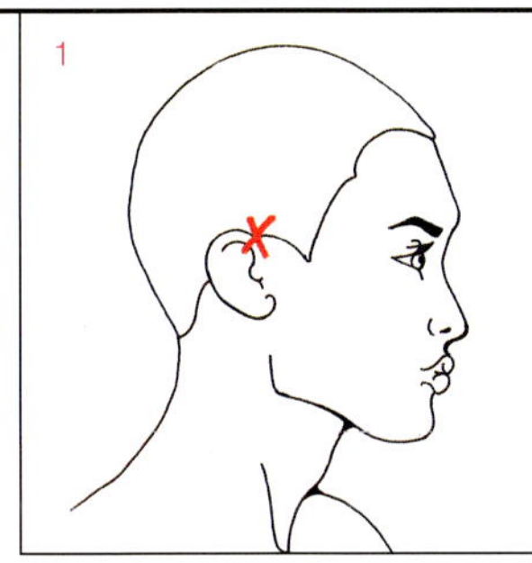

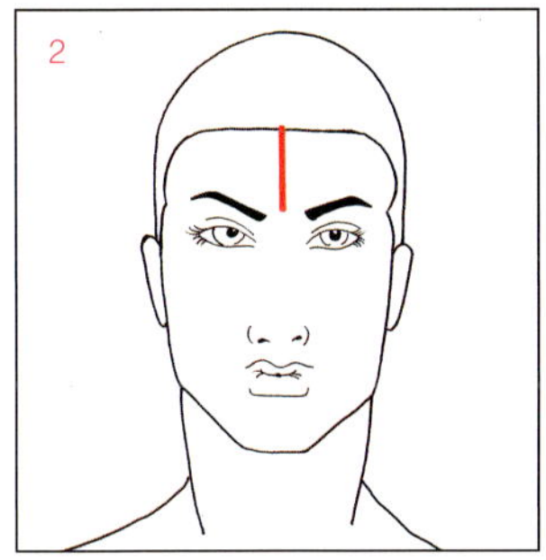

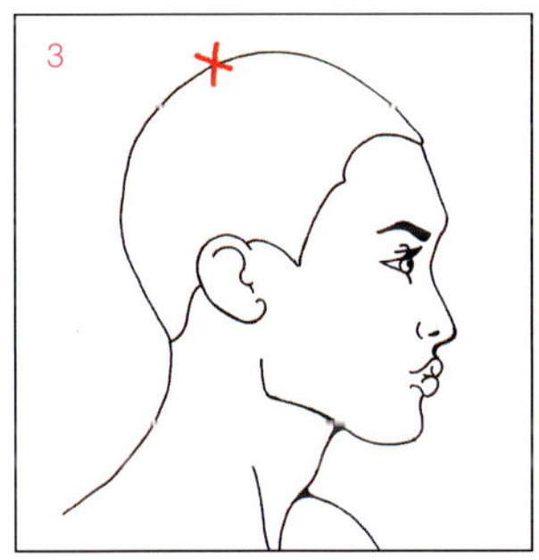

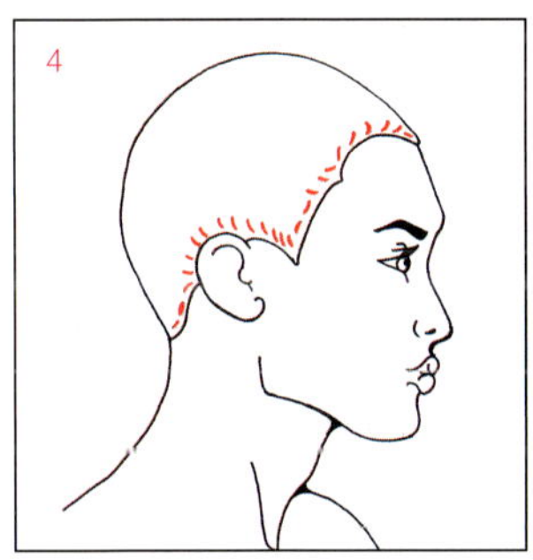

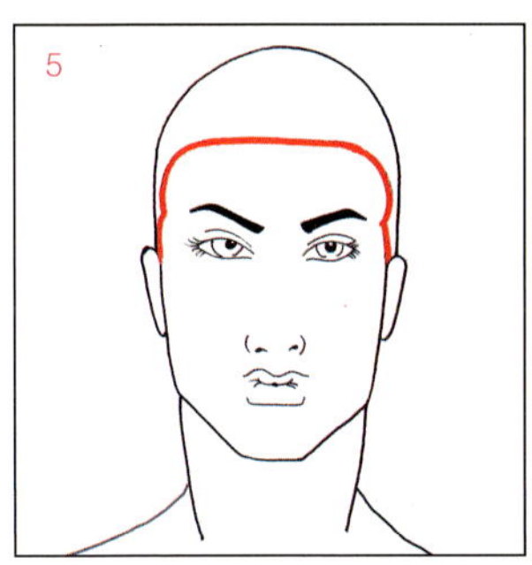

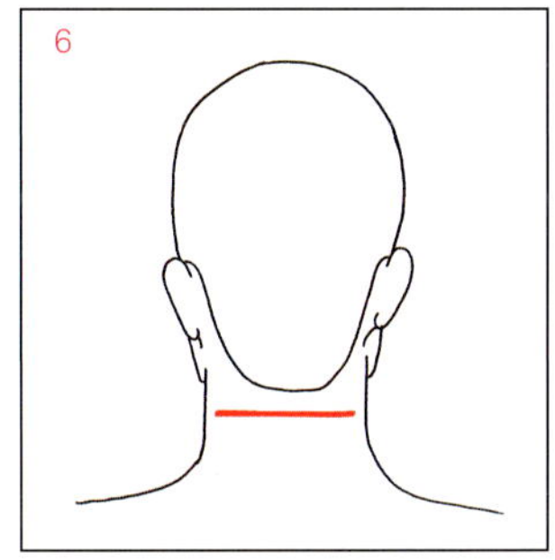

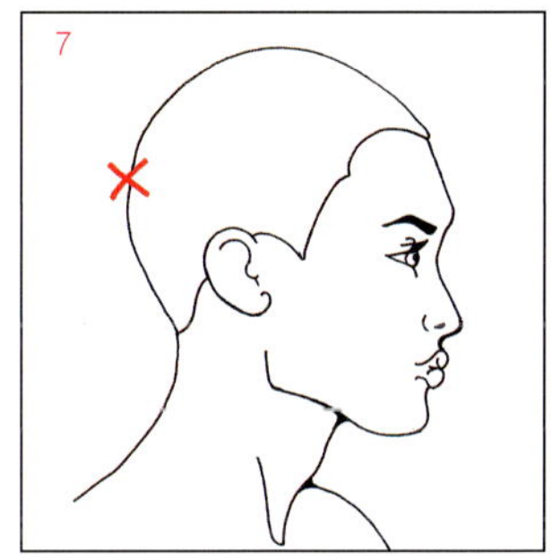

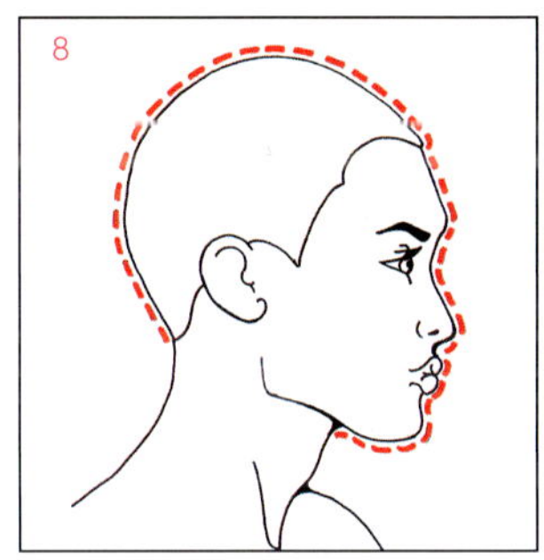

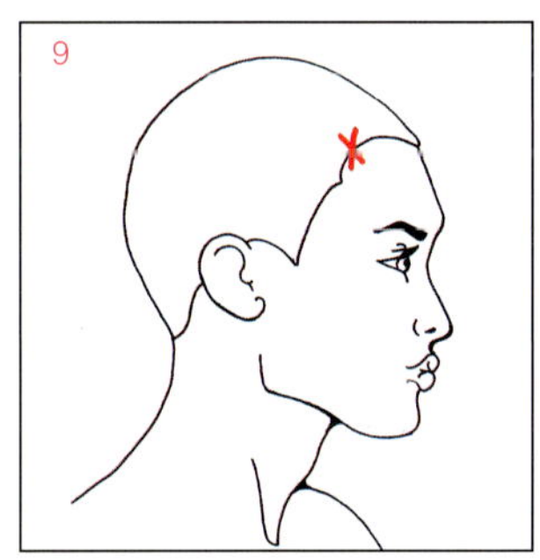

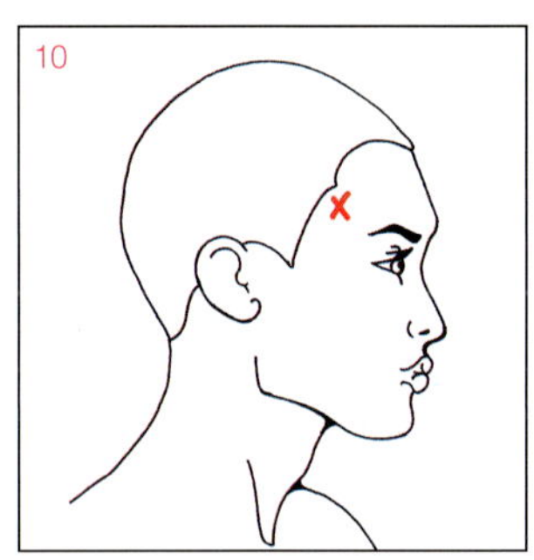

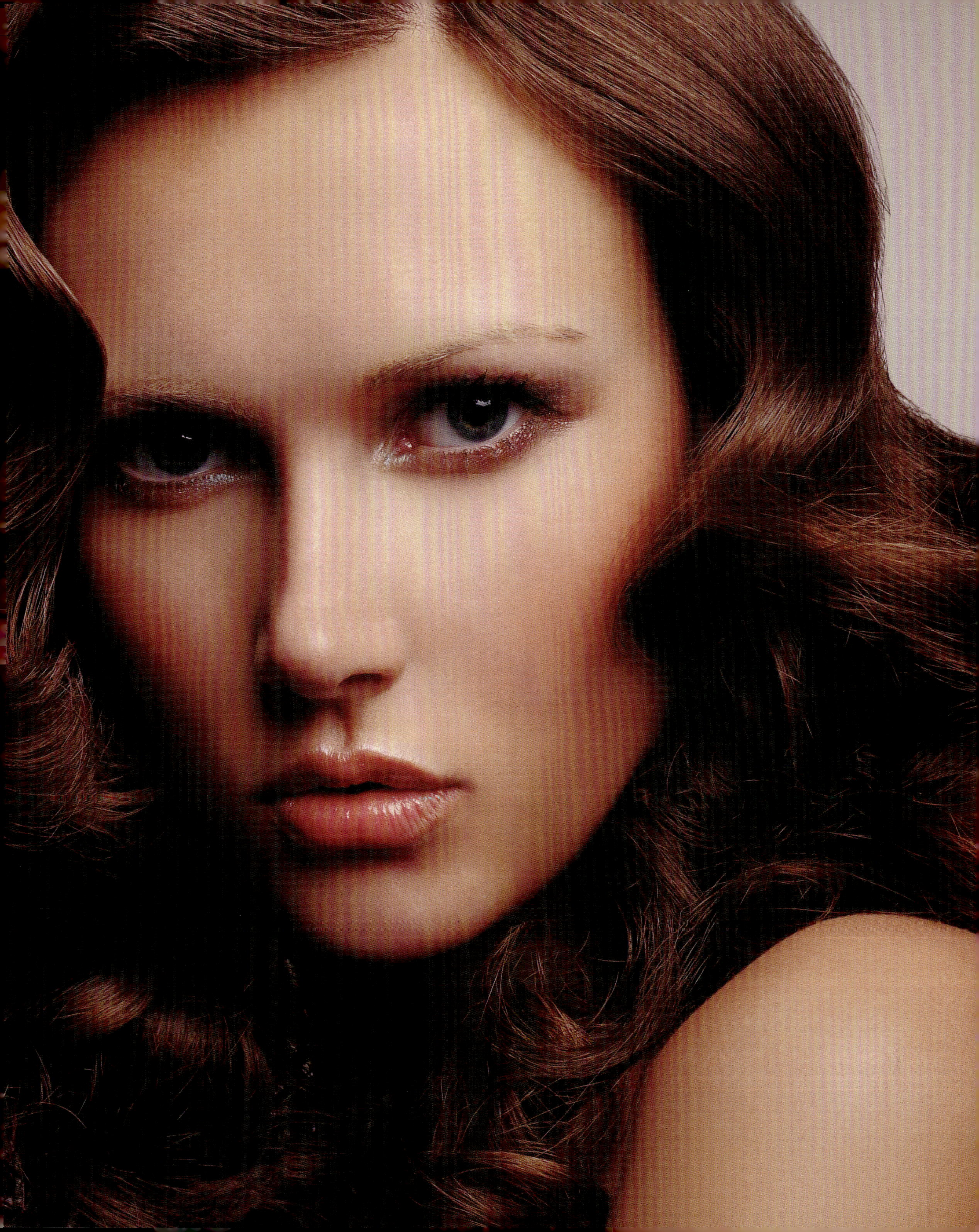

Hair Structure

Human hair has three distinct sections, as detailed below.

The Cuticle This is the protective outer layer of the hair – it's the coating you can feel, and if it becomes damaged it feels rough and the hair feels dry. The cuticle is made up of layers of cells that overlap and look like scales on a fish, or tiles on a roof.

Some shafts of hair can have as many as 11 layers of cuticle cells, while others have fewer – this differs by hair type. When a shaft of hair has many layers of cuticle it may become resistant to chemicals, making it difficult for these chemicals such as colour or perm to penetrate the cuticle and into the cortex to become effective and do their work.

Hair that has damage to the cuticle or has cuticle missing will be porous. The cuticle is colourless and translucent; this means that it lets in light, allowing the cortex to be seen.

The Cortex The cortex is the largest part of the hair; it's the area where all the main chemical changes occur. Natural colour pigments are found in the cortex – these granules of colour pigment are known as melanin.

The cortex consists of long chains of cells that form a spiral into fibres. These fibres spiral together into fibre bundles and groups of these bundles form the inside of the hair. The fibre bundles are held together inside the cortex by different types of bond. The bonds consist of weak salt and hydrogen bonds (these are broken by water or heat), and very strong disulphide bonds that can only be broken by chemicals such as perm lotion or relaxer.

The Medulla The medulla is a part of the hair which is not so important to the hairdresser. It has no effect on any hairdressing processes and is not always present in the hair. Some hair when examined under a microscope shows the medulla in patches – present in some areas and absent in others.

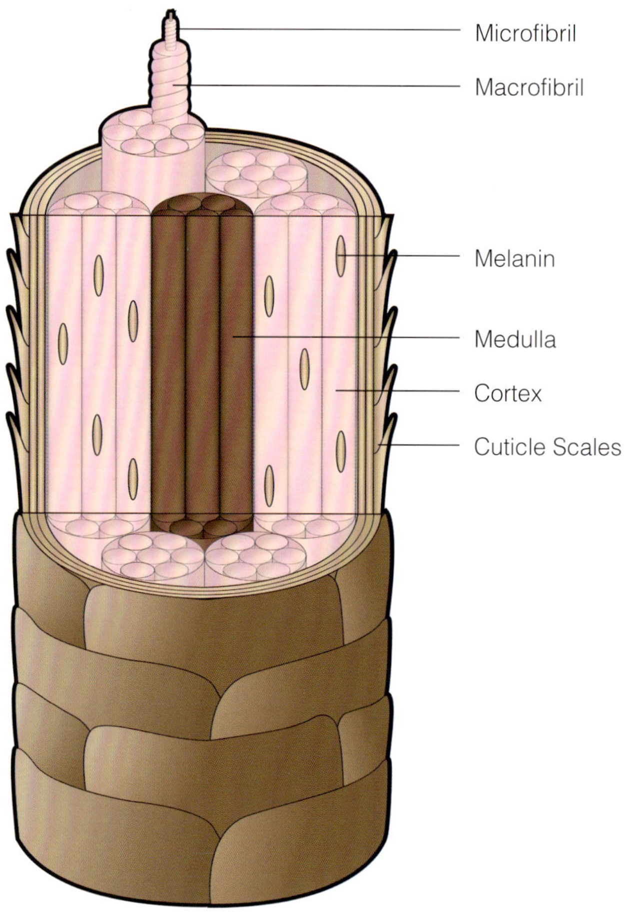
Microfibril
Macrofibril
Melanin
Medulla
Cortex
Cuticle Scales

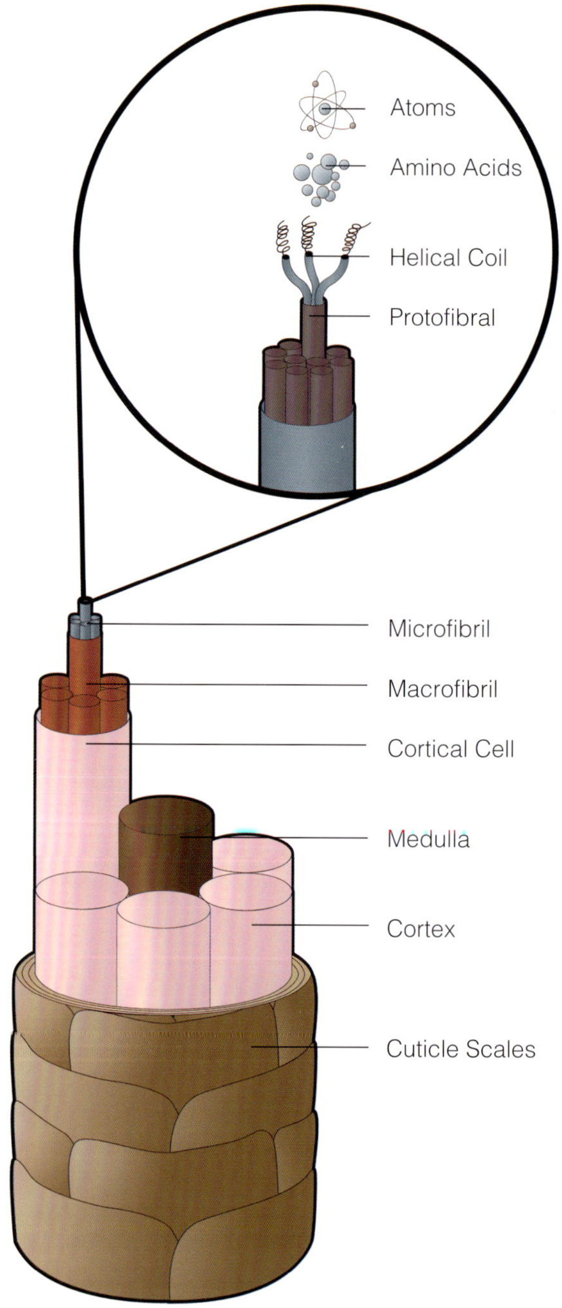
Atoms
Amino Acids
Helical Coil
Protofibral
Microfibril
Macrofibril
Cortical Cell
Medulla
Cortex
Cuticle Scales

The Chemical Structure of Hair

Human hair consists of a hard protein called keratin protein. This protein makes hair elastic and flexible, in turn allowing hair to become stretched, waved, compressed or curled.

Keratin protein is also found in human skin and nails.

Inside the structure of hair you will find atoms that form the beginning of the structure of hair; from these atoms come amino acids. Amino acids combine to form long chains called polypeptides.

Within the hair shaft polypeptides form long chains which look like coiled springs. These springs are held in place by cross-links between the polypeptide chains. There are three types of links – made from sulphur bonds, salt bonds and hydrogen bonds. Together they form disulphide bridges.

Salt and hydrogen bonds are fairly weak and easily broken, which allows the springs to be stretched. This is what happens when heated electrical appliances are used on the hair.

The natural coiled state of keratin is called alpha keratin; when hair has been blow-dried, stretched or set this process creates what is known as beta keratin. This change from alpha to beta keratin is only a temporary one; once the hair becomes wet again it relaxes back to its natural alpha state.

Disulphide bridges are much stronger – they can only be altered during chemical processes such as perming or relaxing. Disulphide bridges give hair its strength.

The composition of hair continues with amino acids binding together to form a helix coil. It usually takes about three helix coils to form a protofibril. A microfibril is composed of around 11 protofibrils. A macrofibril is then formed from the microfibril. These in turn form the cortex; melanin pigments are found in the cortex and give hair its colour.

The medulla occupies the central space within the hair shaft; it is not always present in hair, and even when it's there it serves no useful purpose. Finally the cuticle, the outer layer of the hair shaft made up of colourless translucent scales, covers the hair and forms a protective surface.

To recap, the structure of hair is as follows:

Atoms - Amino Acids - Helix Coil - Protofibril - Microfibril - Macrofibril - Medulla - Cortex - Cuticle.

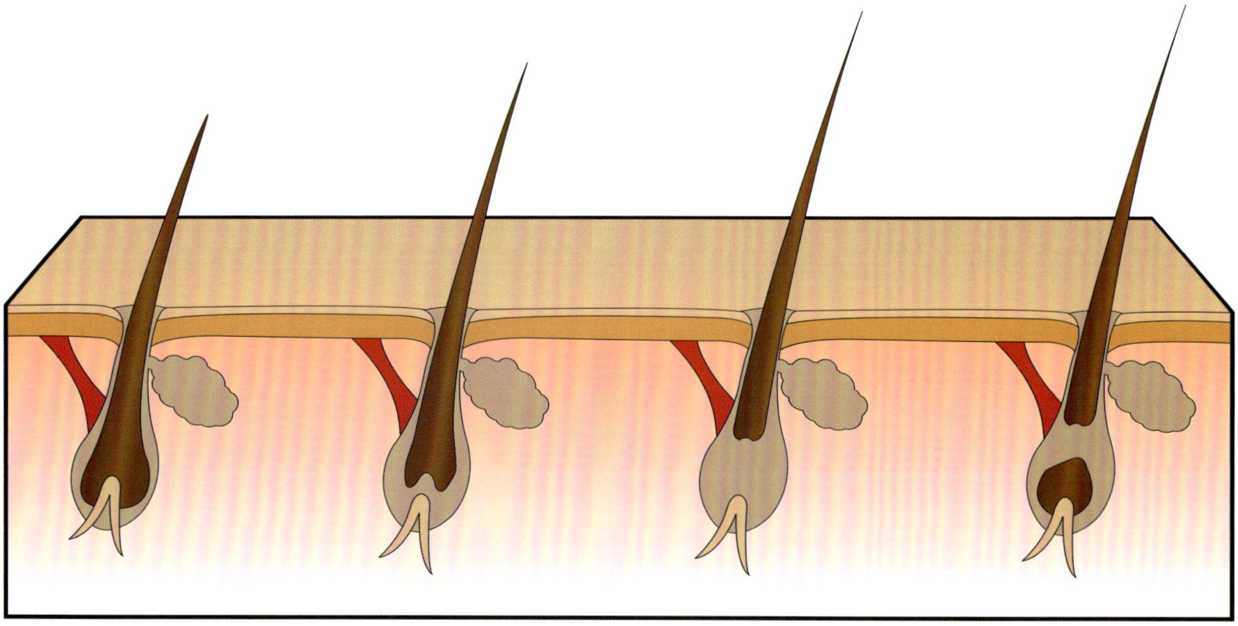

Anagen Catagen Telogen Early Anagen

The Growth Cycle of Hair

Hair grows, stops growing, falls out and then renews itself on a continual basis. If this growth pattern stops or is temporarily halted in some way, and if hair does not replace itself, areas of baldness will appear.

Most human hair grows continually from one to seven years. Some people cannot grow their hair long while others can grow their hair very long – this is because they have an unusually long growing stage in the growth pattern.

There are three stages in the growth cycle:

Anagen
This is the main growing stage when the germinal matrix and the papilla (see p36) are working hard to produce hair cells. This process can last from a few months to a few years.

Catagen
This stage is when the hair stops growing and the hair bulb gradually separates from the papilla and shrinks away from it upwards inside the follicle.

Telogen
This is the resting stage when no growth occurs. The follicle shrinks and fully separates from the papilla. This stage does not usually last very long, generally up to about four months. If it does not come to an end, then baldness results.

The human hair growth cycle is individual to each hair as they reach different stages at different times, so that there is a continuous renewal and replacement of old hairs.

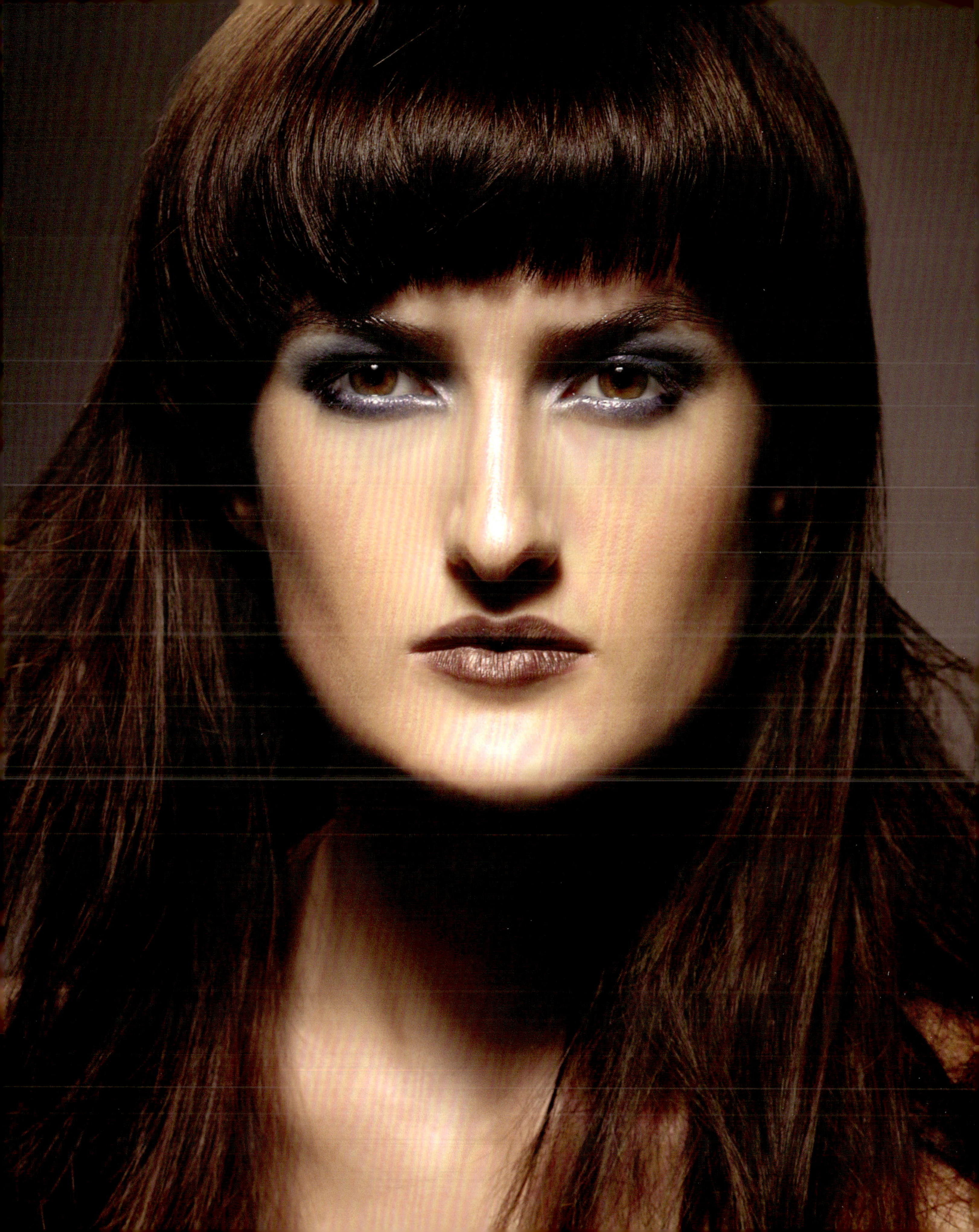

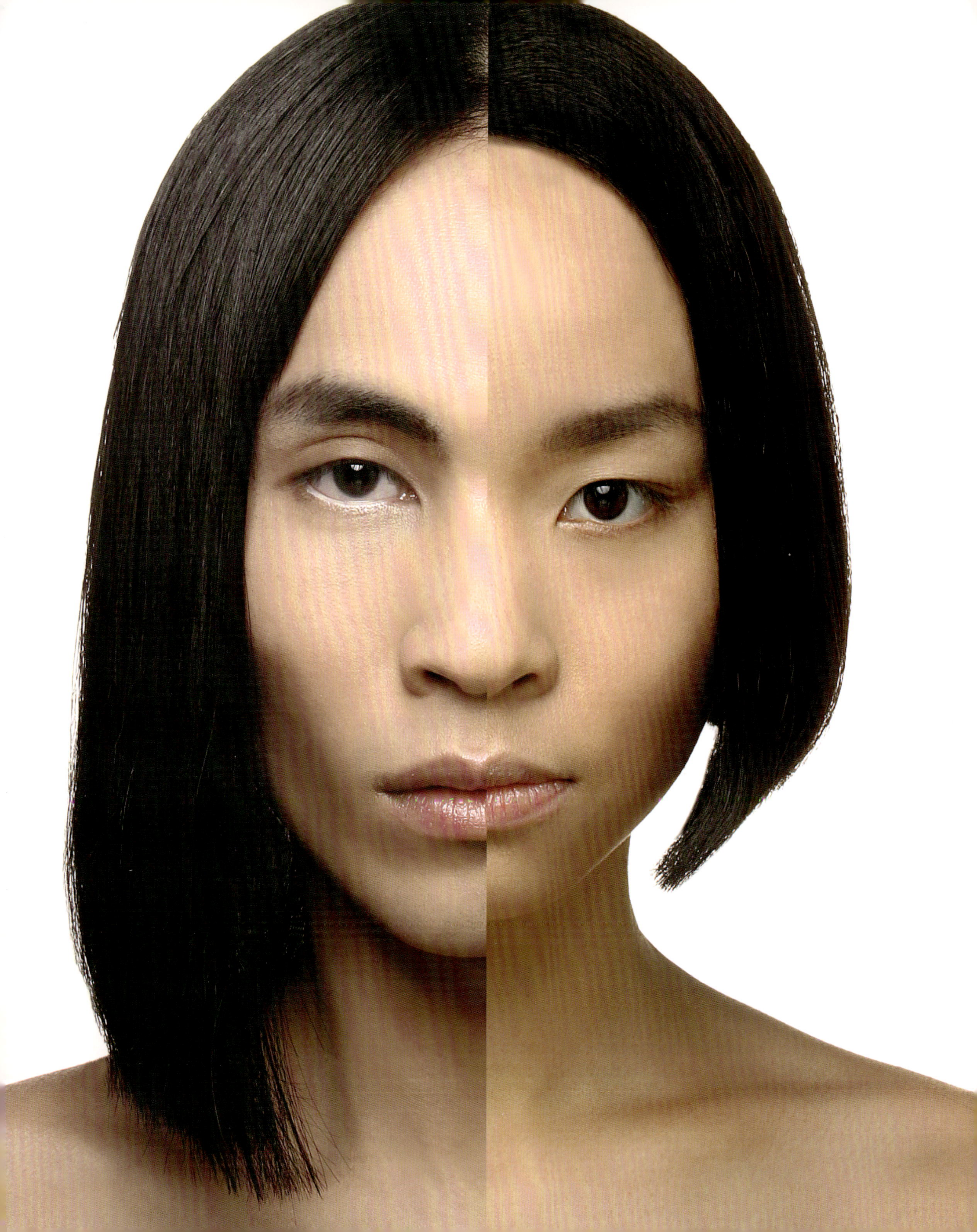

Hair Types and Textures

There are three different types of human hair: European, Asian and Afro-Caribbean.

European or Caucasian hair can be straight, wavy or curly in texture, it also varies in colour from very dark brown to light blonde. When examined under a microscope in a cross-section, it is oval in shape.

Asian hair tends to be straight and limp. When a cross-section is examined under the microscope the shape of the hair is round. This hair type varies in colour from very dark brown to medium brown. Asian hair is often very thick and strong, if it is cut fairly short it sometimes stands straight out from the head.

Afro-Caribbean hair is usually very tightly curled and often very dark in colour. It is very easily damaged and all treatments, especially chemical treatments, must be carried out with care. The shape of the hair when looked at in a cross-section is almost kidney shaped.

Hair texture can be described in the following way: fine, medium or coarse. This means that each hair is fine, medium or thick when looking at the size of its circumference. The circumference defines the texture of the hair. If a hair has a large circumference measurement it is considered to be coarse, if it has a small circumference measurement it has a fine texture.

The density of hair means how many individual hairs there are on any one head. So a fine-textured head of hair may have much more hair than a coarse-textured head of hair. The hair types we have are characteristically hereditary.

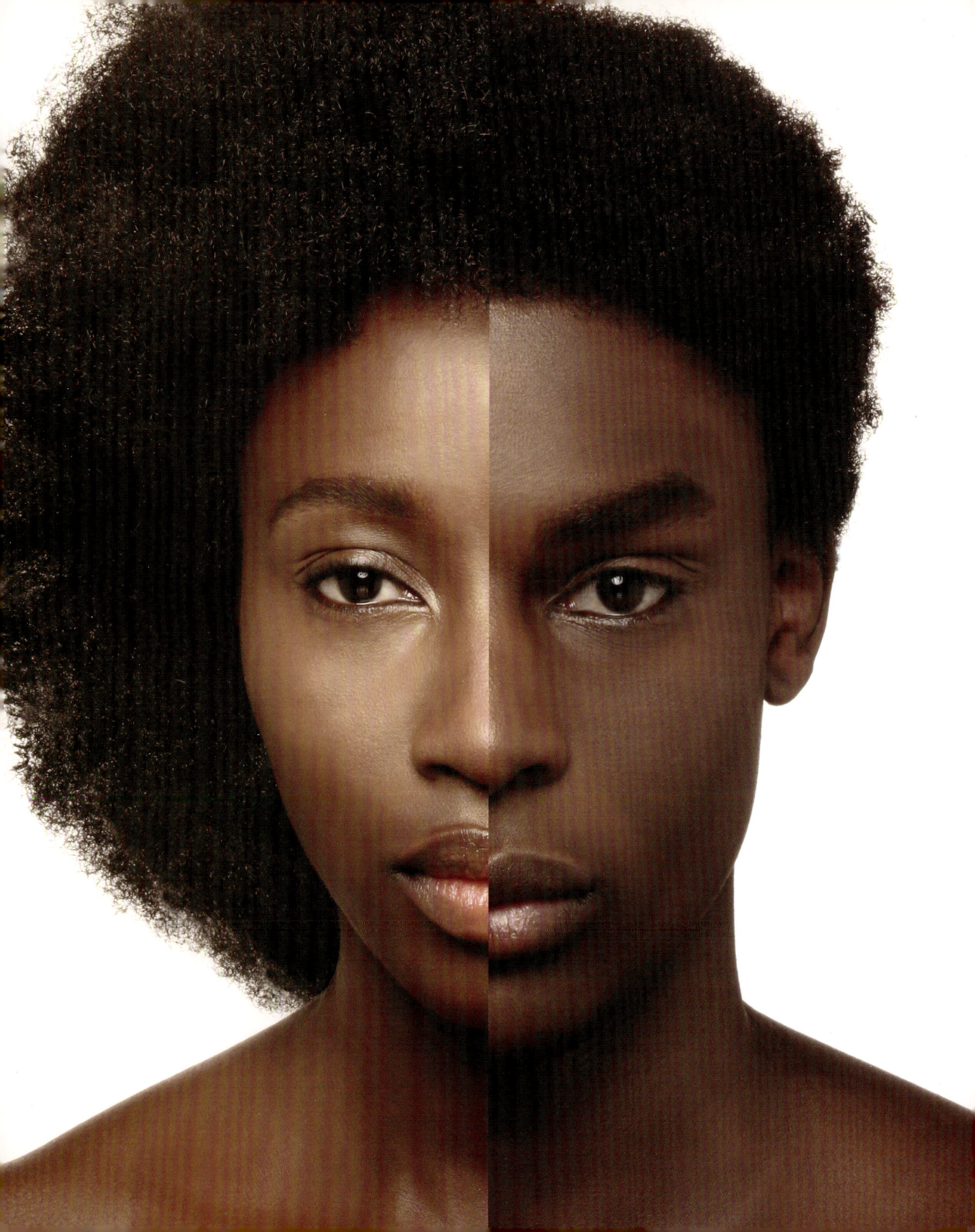

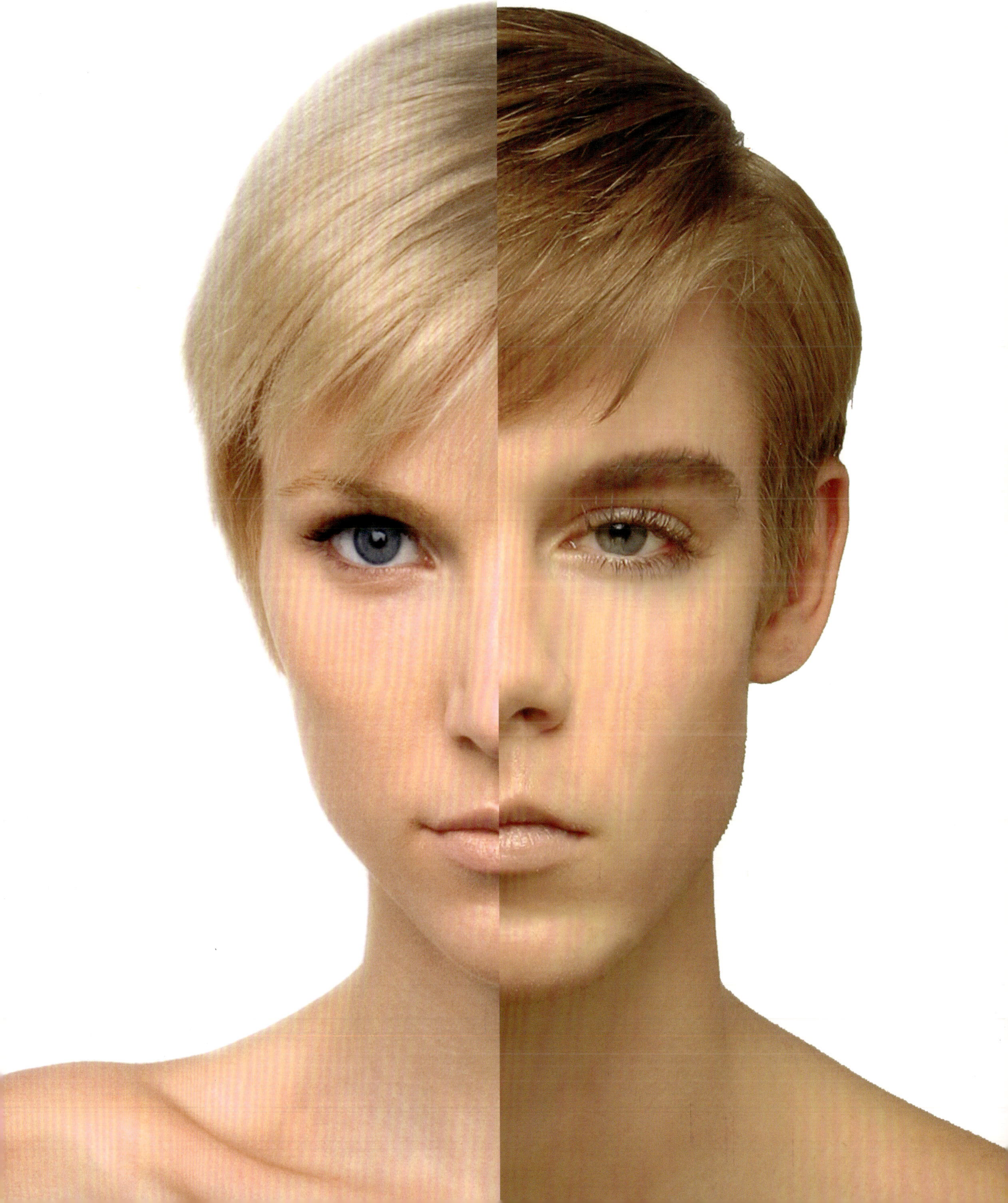

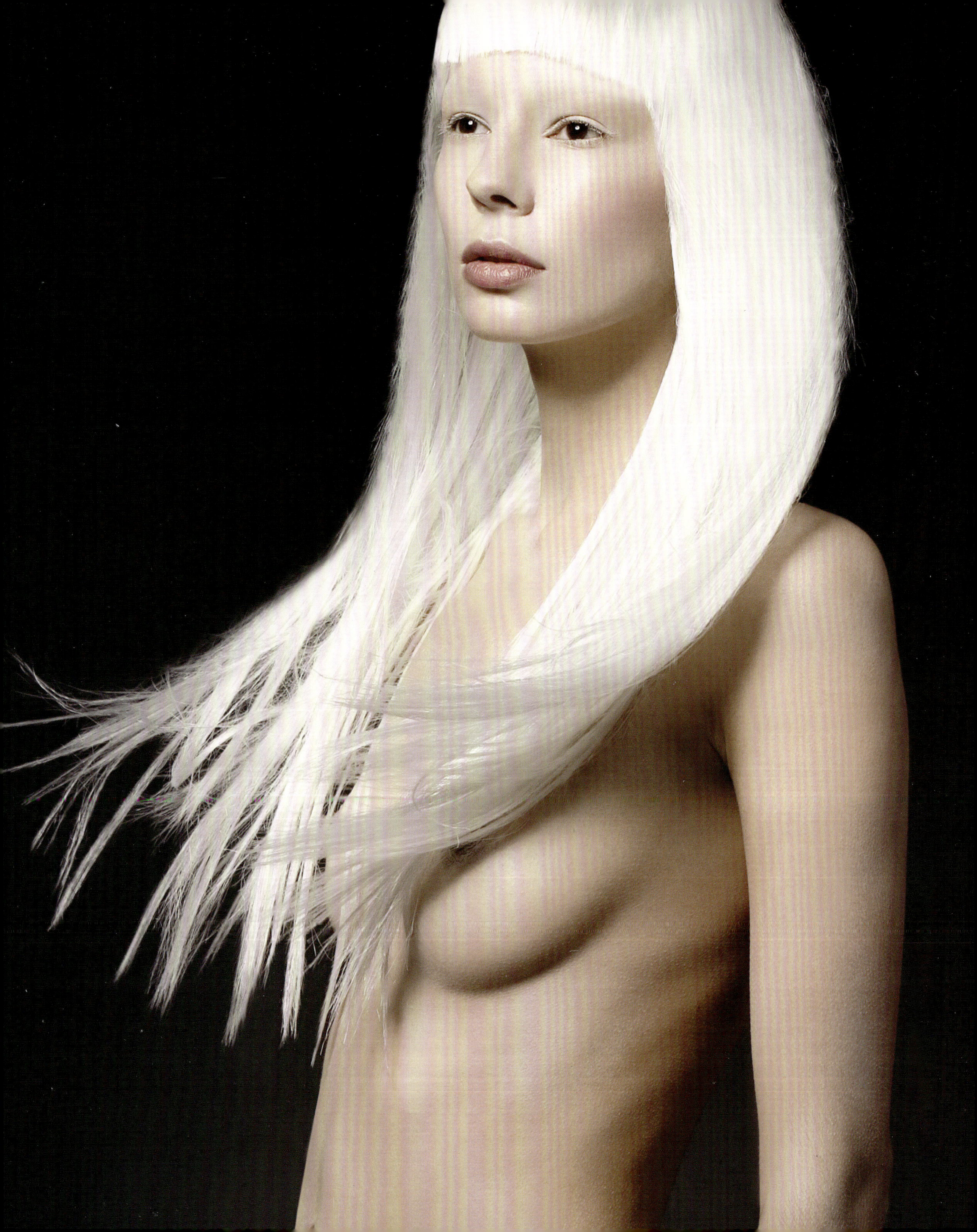

Testing on Hair and Scalp

In hairdressing it is very important to have an understanding of salon procedures and manufacturers' instructions in relation to conducting tests on your clients' hair and scalp. This means knowing how and when tests should be carried out, the importance of doing tests and the potential consequences of failing to do them.

The tests are as follows:

- skin test
- elasticity test
- porosity test
- incompatibility test
- strand test
- pre-colour test

The importance of each test includes knowing:

- when to do it
- how to do it
- why it should be done
- the expected results
- the possible consequences of failing to do it

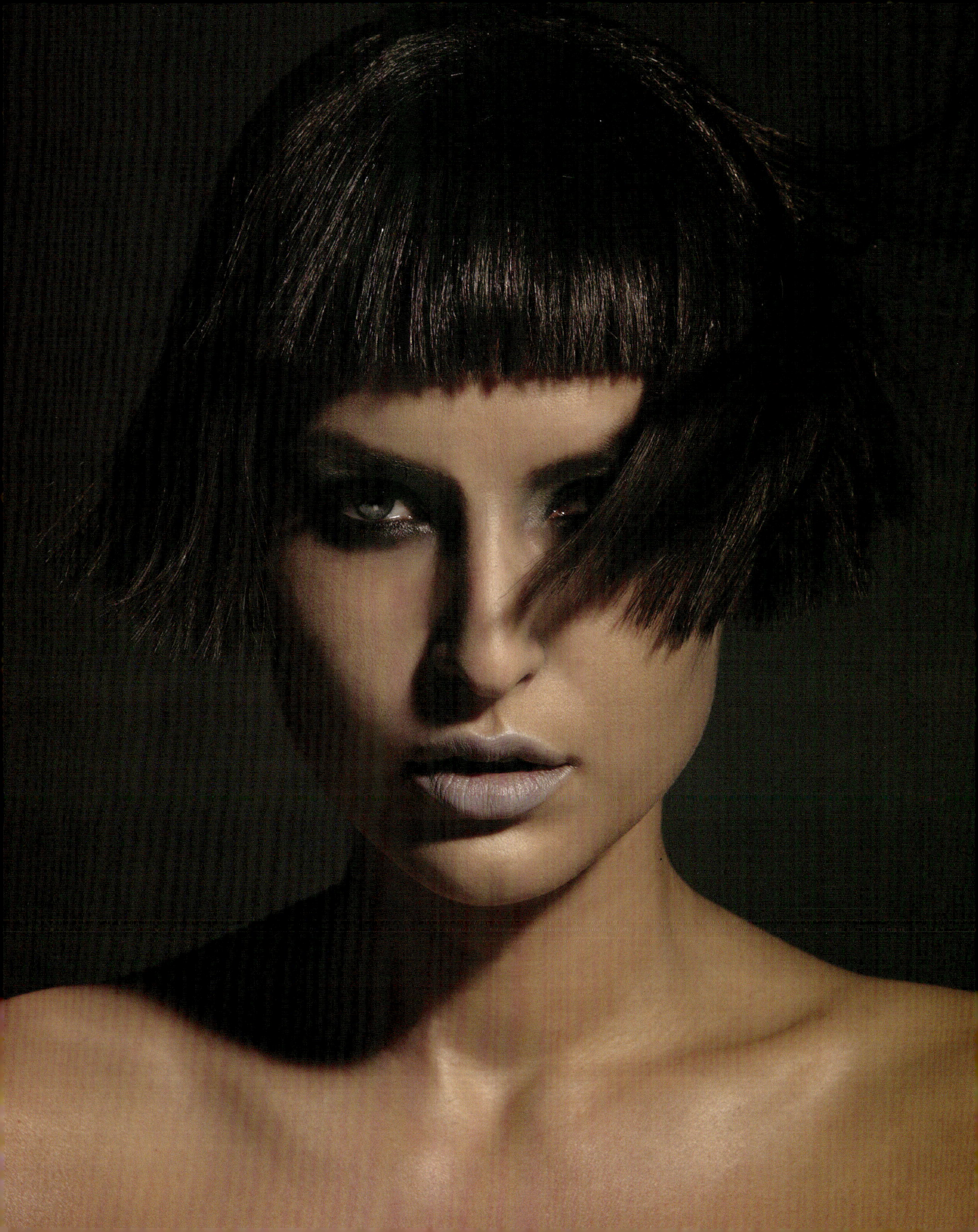

Hair and Skin Tests

Testing is always a good idea, if you are unsure about the outcome of a service; also testing on hair and scalp will help you and your client maintain confidence.

Skin Tests – these are carried out before a client has an on-scalp colour application. The test should be carried out 24 hours before the service. If the client has an allergic reaction symptoms are usually redness, itching and blistering. A substance known as para dye is an ingredient found in permanent hair colour; testing is necessary to find out if a client will have an allergic reaction to it. Under no circumstances should colour be used on the client in the event of an allergic reaction.

Method: apply a small amount of surgical spirit on cotton wool and clean an area behind the ear or in the crease of the elbow. Mix a small amount of colour (the target shade) with equal parts of hydrogen peroxide 6% (20 vol.). Apply a small amount of colour mixture to the cleansed area and allow to dry. Cover with a plaster or collodion (new skin) if available. Ask the client to leave the colour on for 24 hours: tell them that if there is any irritation the colour should be washed off and calamine lotion should be applied to soothe the skin. Record what has been used on the client's skin, together with client details: name, address and date. When your client returns to the salon check the result.

Elasticity Tests – these involve testing the internal strength of hair. When hair is in good condition it is springy and bouncy – this means it has good elasticity. The hair will stretch up to one third its length when dry and half its length when it is wet, and then it will return to its original length. When hair has lost its elasticity this is because bonds in the cortex have been damaged, usually due to over-processing with chemical treatments.

Method: to test hair for elasticity, take a couple of strands of hair and hold between the thumb and forefinger of each hand and pull gently. If the hair stretches more than half its length, then it is over-elastic and could break off, especially during a chemical process. A course of intense conditioning treatments is advisable.

Porosity Tests – these are carried out to test the outer layers of the cuticle. Porous hair can absorb liquids like water or chemicals through the cuticle and into the cortex. When the cuticle lies flat and the hair feels smooth, then the hair is undamaged. If the hair is chemically or physically damaged then it becomes porous or unevenly porous. Any chemical treatments applied to porous hair may result in an uneven curl with a perm or uneven colour results. Acid perm lotions are used for coloured hair, as a normal strength lotion would over-process the hair; also application of colour could become patchy on the hair.

Method: take a strand of hair and hold it by its root with the thumb and forefinger, sliding a finger along the hair travelling from the direction of root to end. If the hair feels rough and bumpy the cuticle is open or missing: this means the hair is porous. If the hair feels smooth then the cuticle is flat and closed and is in good condition.

Incompatibility Tests – some chemicals used in hairdressing do not work together: they are incompatible. For example henna contains metallic salts which are incompatible with other chemicals you may intend to use. Carry out an incompatibility test before perming, colouring or bleaching if you think the hair has a doubtful history.

Method: in a glass container mix together 10ml hydrogen peroxide and 10ml alkaline perm lotion. Take a small slice of hair and place it in the solution and wait a few minutes. If the hair changes colour or the solution fizzes or heat is given off, this is a positive reaction and the hair should not be permed or coloured with any product containing hydrogen peroxide.

Strand Test – this is conducted once any of the following products are on the hair. This is to check the development of colour on the hair ensuring the product has developed thoroughly:

semi-permanent colour
quasi colour
permanent colour
bleach and pre-lightener
colour reducers
relaxer

Method: put on a pair of disposable gloves, then remove some of the product from the hair with the back of a comb or a strip of cotton wool. This will allow you to see if the treatment has developed properly: if you are happy with the result and the process has had full development time, remove product and proceed with service.

Pre-colour Test – a slice of hair is taken, usually underneath the occipital bone, or from any un-noticeable area of the head. This procedure will allow the hair to be tested with any of the following colour products:

temporary colour – coloured setting lotions and coloured mousse
semi-permanent colour – colour which gradually fades
permanent colour – mixed with hydrogen peroxide
bleaches – for full head treatments or highlights and pre-lightening applications

Method: mix a small amount of the product intended for use. Lay the test cutting on a piece of foil and cover the hair with the product. Check manufacturer's instructions for development times: tint and bleach may need longer to develop as there is no heat or warmth coming from the head. Once developed, rinse off. Remember temporary colours are left on the hair. Examine the result. Testing in this way shows whether hair will take colour evenly.

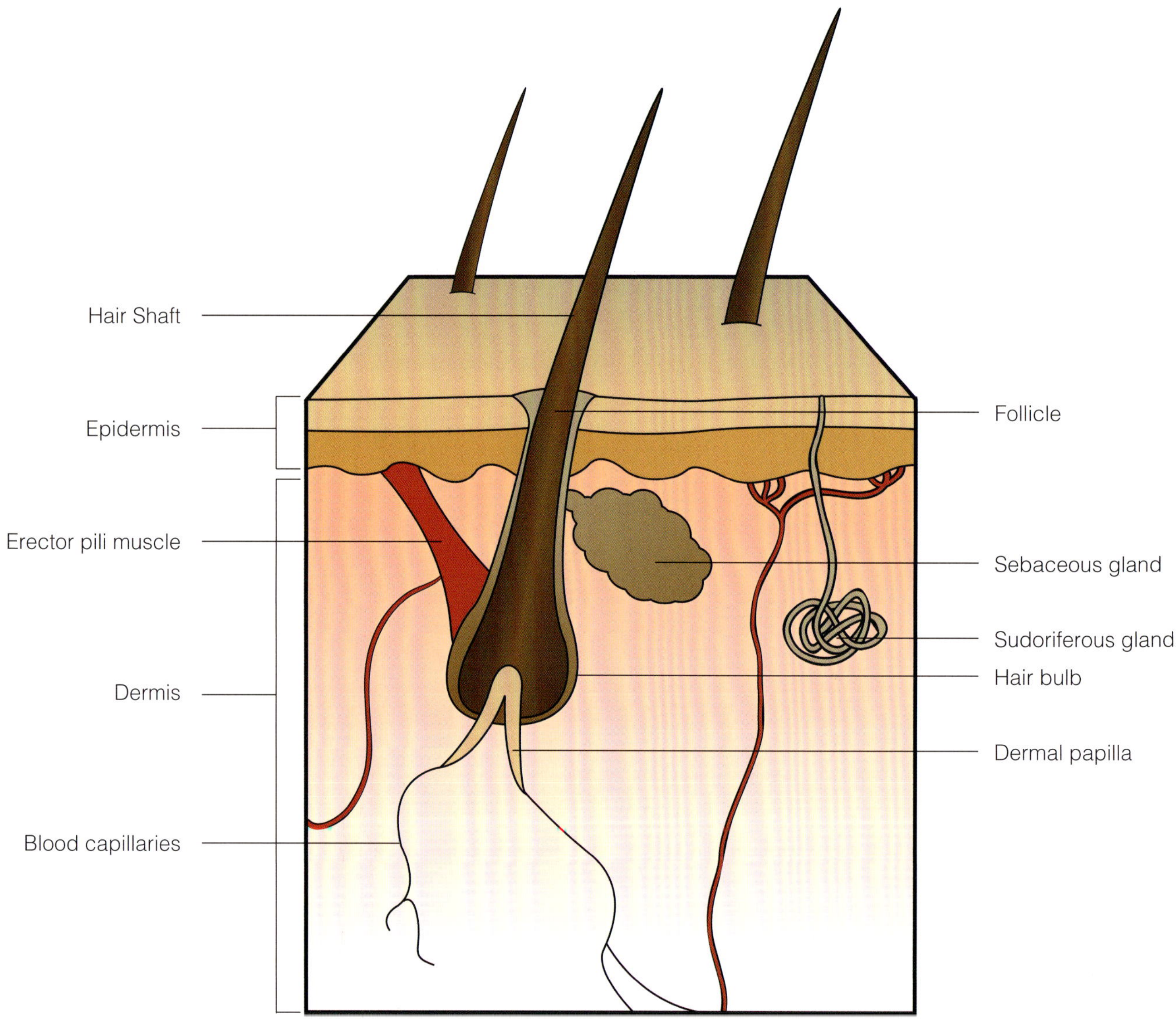
Hair Shaft
Epidermis
Erector pili muscle
Dermis
Blood capillaries
Follicle
Sebaceous gland
Sudoriferous gland
Hair bulb
Dermal papilla

Skin Structure

There are two main layers to skin: the epidermis – this is the surface layer of the skin, the one which we can see and feel; and the dermis – this is a deep layer that has the blood and nerve supply, and is where the hair follicle lies.

The area beneath the dermis is called the subcutaneous layer. This is where the skin stores fat that gives us smooth curves rather than sharp angles.

As well as having a good blood and nerve supply, the skin has various appendages and most of these lie in the dermis. The main appendages are:

The follicles – hair grows through the follicle.
The dermal papilla – all cell growth and cell division of hair occurs here.
The sebaceous gland – this secretes oil called sebum, this protects us against bacteria, as it is slightly acidic; it also lubricates and waterproofs the skin.
The sudoriferous glands – also known as sweat glands, they excrete waste in the form of sweat, which cools the body.
The erector pili muscles – they are attached to the hair follicles. When we are cold the muscles contract: this pulls the hair upright, makes goose pimples and traps warm air from around the body to help keep us warm.

The skin is one of the largest organs of the body and has several main functions:

1. To protect us from strong sunlight and bacteria.
2. There are nerves in the skin that give us sensation – the sense of touch.
3. Glands in the skin transport waste to the surface and also produce oil that waterproofs us.
4. To help to control body temperature: by the evaporation of sweat to cool us and trapping air around us to keep us warm.

The natural pigment of skin and hair is called melanin and is produced by cells called melanocytes.

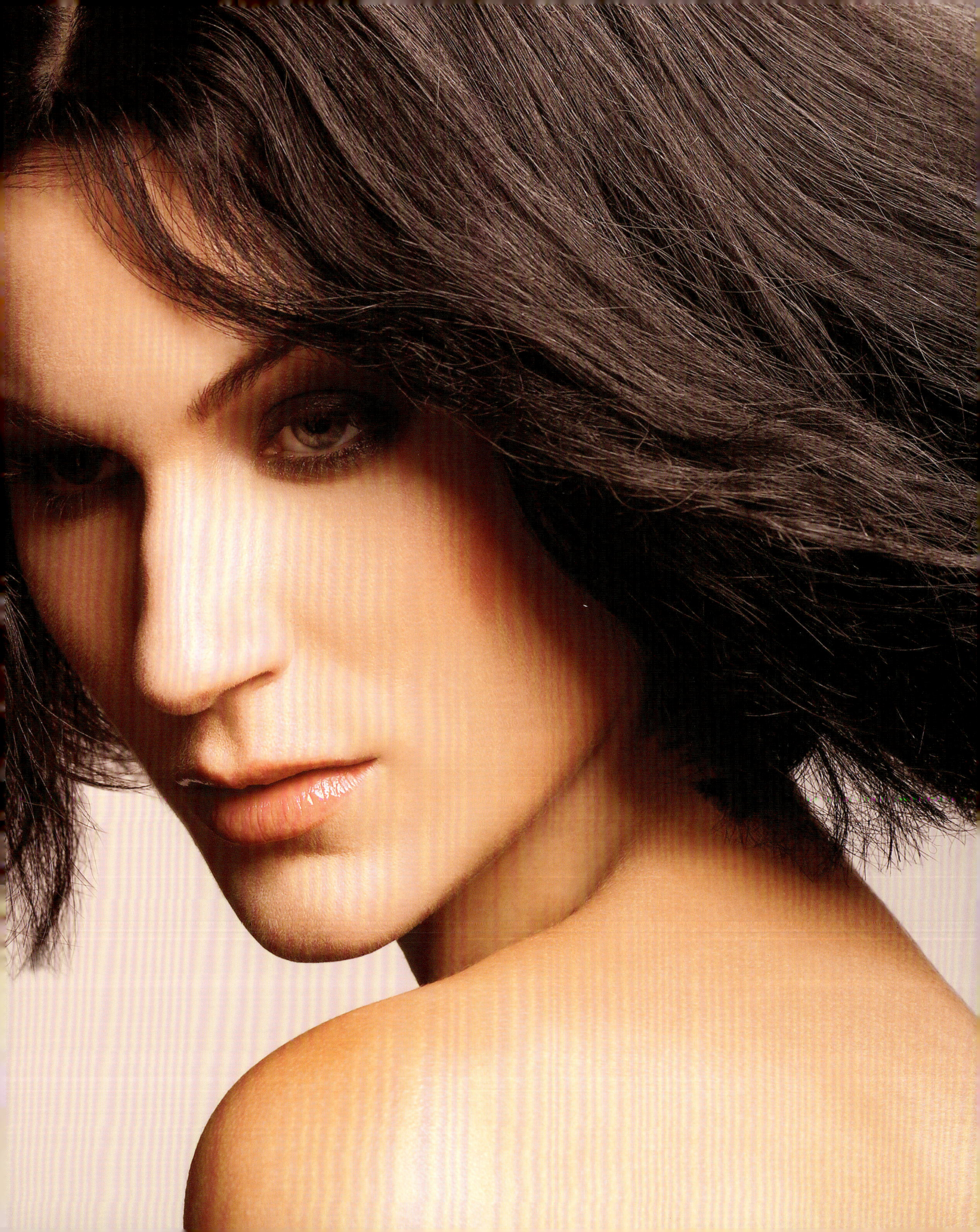

Analysis of Hair and Scalp

During your consultation with your client you will be analysing the hair and scalp and taking into account the following factors:

Porosity – check the condition of the cuticle: is there a smooth or rough feeling to the hair?

Texture – how thick is each individual hair? This depends on the number of layers of cuticle and whether there is a medulla present.

Density – the amount of hair the client has: is there an abundance or is the hair quite sparse?

Length of hair – is the hair very long? Long hair may have been treated many times, it may have undergone many chemical processes.

Growth patterns – it is important to consider the directional growth of the hair, as this will have an effect on the finished result.

Movement – is there any curl or natural movement in the client's hair, has the hair been permed?

Elasticity – hair in good condition is springy and bouncy: hair with poor elasticity will overstretch and snap, for example by chemical over-processing.

Face shape – the shape of the client's face is very important when considering a hairstyle: suitability is key.

Previously treated – are there any chemicals on the hair, such as colour, perm or relaxer? Assess correctly or there may be serious consequences.

Head shape – it is important to take into account the shape of the client's head, not only from the front and back but also the profile.

Lifestyle – create a hairstyle that suits the needs of the client. Take into account the client's personality. Versatility is important: the shape needs to be suitable.

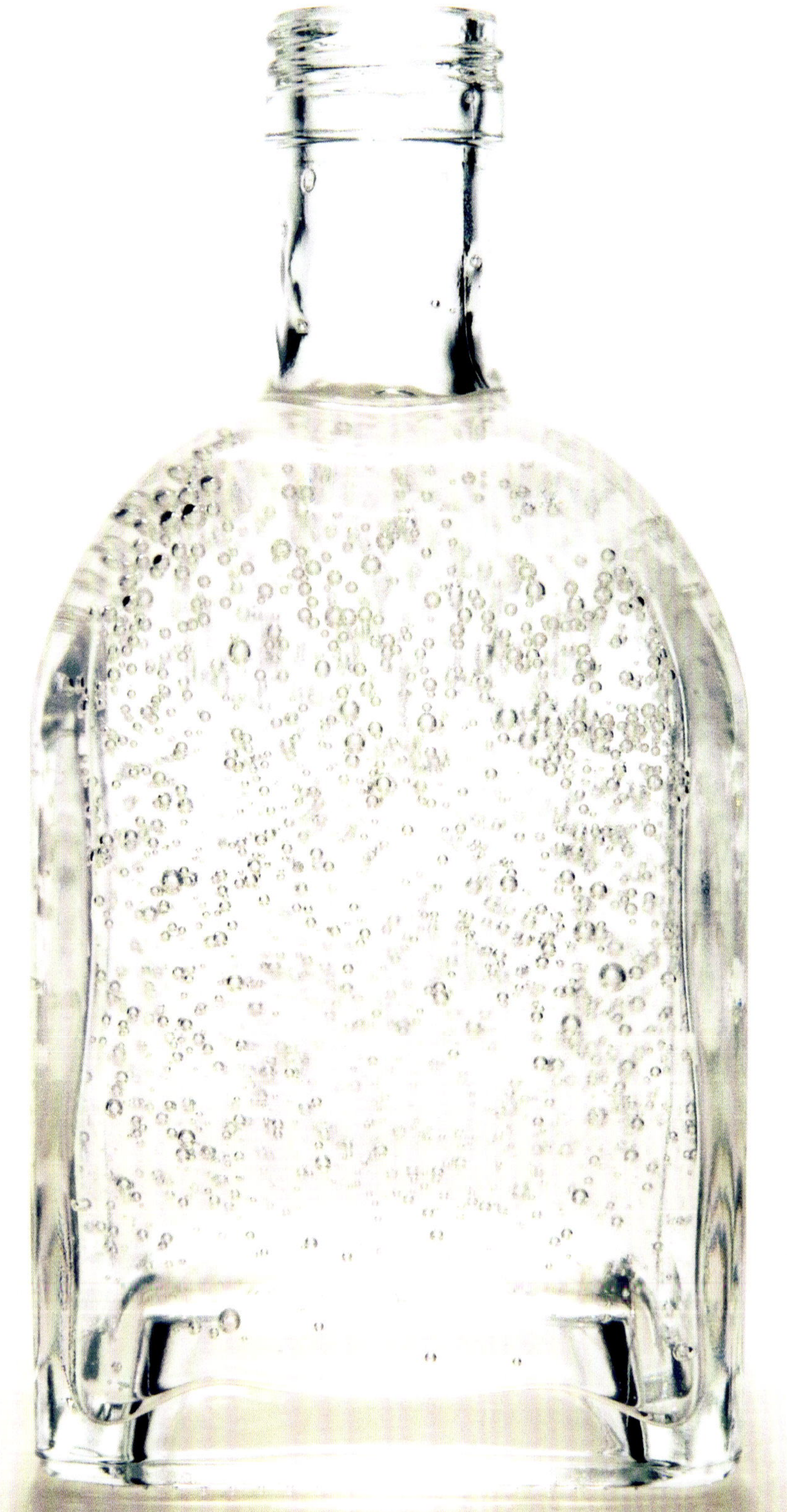

Hair Care

The main aim in hairdressing is for the hairdresser to achieve excellence in cutting, colouring and styling. However this would be incomplete without a correct hair care regime. The secret of beautiful hair relies as much upon conditioning as it does upon excellent cutting. If the hair is in top condition, the finished result will look better and last longer.

Maintaining healthy, shiny hair involves using the correct shampoo. The shampoo should be acid or pH balanced as these products will leave the hair and scalp in the required, slightly acid state. Today's modern shampoos employ various conditioning and moisturising agents to compensate for the deep cleansing action of the shampoo. Hydrolysed wheat and micronised B-5 proteins are examples of excellent materials which penetrate into and act upon the hair giving it additional body and strength.

Shampoo should be used in small quantities, with sufficient activity to cleanse the hair. If there are lasting suds during the first application, this will demonstrate that all styling products and grime have been totally emulsified and that there is still additional activity in the shampoo and one application is sufficient. Only if the suds disappear rapidly is a second shampoo necessary. All traces of shampoo must be rinsed away thoroughly. Residue from shampoo is not recommended and many 'dandruff' complaints are the result of insufficient rinsing. Shampoo which has been left in the hair can cause dryness on the scalp and have a greasy and limp effect on the hair.

Damaging agents affecting the hair include chemical processing, illness, sun, improper or over-frequent blow drying, straightening irons, tongs and other heated appliances, heat, water and of course the increasing age of the hair itself. Liquid Hydrolysed Protein is the finest known reconditioner for damaged hair, both internally and externally. A small amount of this substance, when applied, actually becomes part of the hair itself. Properly acidified (pH 6.0), a liquid protein conditioner not only strengthens the hair shaft, but smooths the cuticle of the hair, restoring lustre and sheen. In effect it fills in the damaged areas of the hair shaft. After conditioning all excess product not absorbed should be thoroughly rinsed away. No client will thank you for leaving his or her hair in a sticky, lacklustre condition.

Conditioning treatments can be used in the form of protein packs. Micronised proteins are absorbed by the hair and protective moisturisers coat the hair, creating super sheen, plus protection against the harsh action of hairdryers and hot irons etc. Treatments are usually used when the hair is in a severely damaged condition with dry and frizzy ends and/or breakage. Two or three treatments are usually necessary to restore the hair to good condition, and from time to time this service should be carried out professionally at the salon. It is important for the client to understand that one treatment cannot work miracles.

As with health and diet, a regime of continuous care is needed to achieve and maintain the desired results. Implementing this will achieve beautiful and healthy-looking hair for your client and be a perfect advertisement for you and your salon.

It is very important that the client understands that a home hair care maintenance programme should be followed to keep the hair in its luxurious condition. The same super quality shampoo should be used in conjunction with conditioners, a frequent conditioning regime should become part of the client's own programme to maintain sheen and healthy hair.

A regular haircut will remove dead, split ends and the untidy effect of irregular growth. It will emphasise the exact shape of the cut or the swinging movement of the hair, which should be as thick at the ends as it is at the roots.

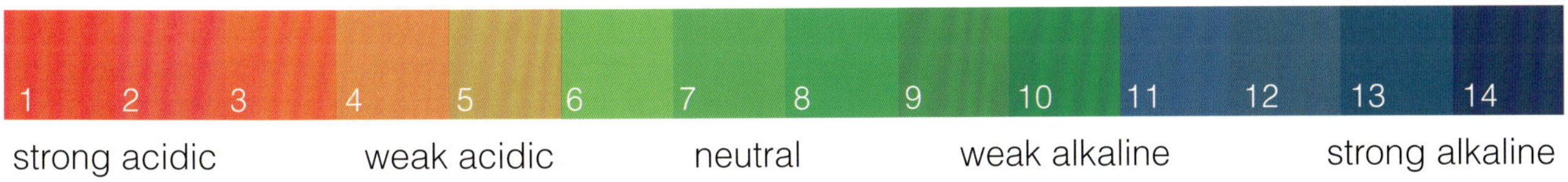

The pH Scale

Most substances have a pH level ranging from 0 to 14. The pH, meaning the potential of hydrogen, measures acidity and alkalinity. Water, for example, has a pH of 7, so is neutral. Zero to six measures acidity and eight to 14 measures alkalinity. The pH value of human hair, skin and nails is around 4.5 to 5.5. Products used in hairdressing such as shampoos and conditioners ideally should be acid balanced, which will maintain the acid mantle of the hair, thus leaving the hair in a slightly acid state and in perfect condition. Products with a pH higher than 7 are likely to be more alkaline and harmful to hair. Using products on the hair that are pH or acid balanced will keep the cuticle closed, giving shine and lustre to hair. But using products that are alkaline will open up the cuticle, making the hair look dull and in poor condition.

Some chemical services in hairdressing such as tinting, pre-lightening, perming and relaxing are high in alkalinity. The reason is that these products need to raise the cuticle layer in order to penetrate the hair shaft and perform the chemical process. To maintain healthy hair and scalp, recommend that your client uses shampoos and conditioners that are acid balanced to keep their hair in top condition.

Maintaining Healthy Hair

The main factors in maintaining healthy hair are:

Health

When you are healthy this will be reflected in your skin and hair. A key factor in ensuring good health is a good diet and enough exercise. A balanced diet consisting of enough fresh fruit and vegetables, sufficient protein and carbohydrates and plenty of clean water will maintain good health.

If you take regular exercise it helps to maintain good circulation that in turn will carry nutrients to the hair follicles. If the body is suffering from an illness, this will be reflected in the condition of the skin and hair – hair could become limp and unmanageable.

Environment

Your surroundings have an impact on how healthy your hair and skin look and feel. If you live in an area where the pollution levels are high, your hair will become coated with these impurities and will need to be cleansed and conditioned on a daily basis. If you live close to the sea then salt which is present in the air will have the same effect. Some areas of the country have soft water and others have hard water. This will have a strong influence on your hair and also on the shampoos and conditioners you should use.

Chemicals

Every time you apply a chemical to hair, some damage is done to it. Certain chemicals are more damaging than others. Permanent colour, a chemical commonly used in hairdressing, is the least damaging; this is followed by mild acidic perm solution, going up to the stronger chemicals used on hair like very alkaline perm solution, then onto bleach and finally to chemical straighteners and relaxers.

Basic Products

Shampoo

Moisturising
For naturally dry hair and chemically distressed hair

Gentle Cleansing
For fine flyaway hair and frequent use

Deep Cleansing
For oily hair and scalp or for swimmers – removes chlorine

Treatment
For chemically distressed hair that requires essential moisture

Scalp
To ease the problem of flaky and itchy scalp

Condition

Surface
For normal to dry hair – repairs broken cuticles

Leave-in
Designed to work on all hair types, excellent de-tangler

Deep Penetration
For hair that is extremely chemically distressed and needs re-building

Treatment
Gives long-term conditioning and repair to increase internal strength

Peppermint/Tea Tree
Stimulates the scalp, invigorating scalp rub

Style

Heat Protection
Thermo protection spray designed for use when blow drying hair

Straightening Balm
Used on damp hair when blow drying, smooths and adds shine

Mousse
For volume and hold, use on wet hair when blow drying and setting

Gel
For use on wet or dry hair, gives lasting hold and control

Curl Activator
Spray or cream, use on damp hair and diffuse for curl definition

Finish

Paste
Ideal for a matt, textured finish – gives support and hold, use on dry hair

Pomade
A water-based non-greasy product, smooths out and adds shine to hair

Hairspray
Finish and fix hair in place with hairspray – some sprays contain UV protection

Shine Spray
Spray a light mist of shine spray onto dry, styled hair for added gloss

Wax/Texturisers
Use for definition and texture, gives a rough finish and solid hold

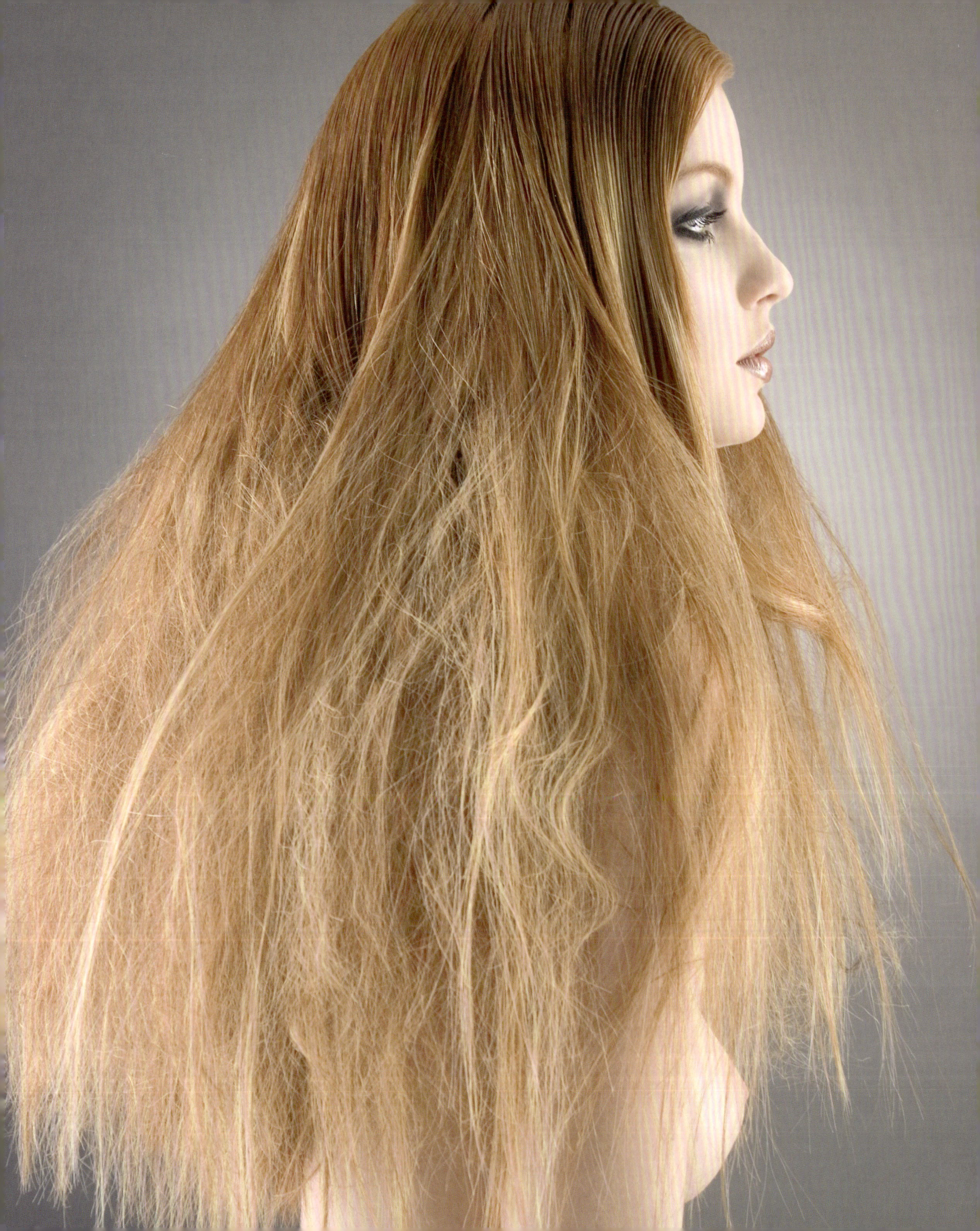

Consultation

In hairdressing it is very important to have a good rapport with your clientele as this will determine your success as a hairdresser. Hairdressers are usually excellent communicators and the relationship between the stylist and client is built on quality of service. This means being a professional, trustworthy and a good listener, all of which are important factors. Good communication ensures effectiveness in the salon: however poor communication can lead to misunderstandings, misinterpretation and mistakes.

Client consultation means talking to your client and giving advice to a client prior to starting work on their hair. During the consultation you will also be examining your client's hair and scalp. By brushing through, you will be able to diagnose any hair or scalp conditions and make appropriate recommendations, for example advising on shampoo and conditioner.

Next, find out what the client wants in accordance with the service they have requested.

When discussing a service with a client, it is important that you ask open-ended questions. These questions usually start with what, how, why, when and where. These types of questions do not allow the client to answer with a straightforward yes or no, they open up a topic for discussion.

Clients may have no idea of what they want to have done to their hair. This is your opportunity to make recommendations and to build up a good relationship with your client. With experience you will be able to produce a perfect hairstyle for each individual client by considering the following: face shape, height and size of the client, age and occupation, lifestyle and personality.

Giving a client accurate information on a hairstyle may lead to further appointments and will promote a professional salon image. Offer all clients a free consultation. Your communication skills are just as important when working with new clients as they are with regular clients. Smiling encourages friendliness and a pleasant atmosphere.

Contraindications

A contraindication is a condition that is present usually on the client's hair or scalp. It is often something that will limit a salon service. If a contraindication is present this means that a service should not be carried out at all. A service may be unsuitable because a client has a medical condition which may be external and visible, or it could be hidden and later discovered in the consultation. Here are some reasons why a client's contraindication may limit a service:

A symptom could be contagious, meaning there is a risk of cross-infection to the stylist and to other clients: for example in the case of head lice.

A client's condition may be made worse by a service: for example open cuts or sores on the client's scalp, later causing irritation.

There may be a reaction to a service which puts the client's health at risk: for example an allergic reaction to colour.

Look at your client in the mirror, or face to face. Eye contact can express friendliness and trust and shows that you are paying attention. Listen to your client. Many clients never return to a salon because, although they have been given a fabulous new hair-style, it was not the one they asked for.

Speak to your client and explain any reasons for delays straightaway and in a polite manner. Always be honest and factual. If the client is rushed for time or appears rather cross then ask your salon manager for help.

Before starting work, always check that the client has removed large earrings, or other jewellery (necklaces and glasses) if necessary before gowning up. Ask the client to keep their valuables in a safe place (in a bag or at reception). Allow enough time to complete your consultation.

All the above should be done before gowning up your client. Gowns should always be freshly laundered and tied securely. Make sure you tuck the client's clothing inside the gown.

Clean towels should be used for every client and must be placed securely around the client's neck. Make sure that your working area is clean and tidy and free from hair. All your tools should be cleaned and sterilised before use. You should make sure that your posture is correct and also that of your client. Try to maintain high standards and a good level of consistency in your work. Finally always try and present yourself to others as a true professional, as first impressions count.

Service	Hair Type	Hair Texture	Hair Density	Scalp	Face Shape
Cut	Afro	Fine	Fine	Normal	Oval
Blow-dry	Asian	Medium	Medium	Dry	Round
Colour	European	Coarse	Thick	Greasy	Square
Perm		Curly		Flaky	Heart
Relaxer		Wavy			Pear
Set		Straight			Oblong
Hair-up					

Previous Treatments	Testing	Hair Growth Patterns	Hair Length	Present Condition
Perm	Porosity	Cow's lick	Above shoulders	Virgin
Relaxer	Elasticity	Double crown	Below shoulders	Chemically treated
Permanent tint	Incompatibility	Widow's peak	One length	Dry
Quasi	Skin	Nape whorls	Layered	Normal
Semi-permanent	Strand		With fringe	Porous
Temporary colour			Without fringe	
Bleach				

Product Recommendation	The Cut	Barbering	Cutting Techniques	Drying Techniques	Setting Techniques
Shampoo	The One Length Cut	Stretch Graduation	Club/blunt	Power dry	Roller
Conditioner	The Classic Bob	Round Layers	Point	Finger dry	Rod
Conditioning treatment	Forward Graduation	Square Graduation	Texturising	Brush and blow dry	Tong
Styling products	The Graduated Bob	Interpretation	Scissor over comb	Attachment	Finger wave
Finishing products	Square Layers	Clipper		Interpretation	Pin-curls
	Round Layers	Razor			Heated rollers
	Concaved Layers				Interpretation
	Square Graduation				
	Intorprotation				

Hair-up	Colour	Application	Permanent Wave/ Relaxer
Pony tail	Temporary	Full head/partial colour	Acid
Chignon	Semi-permanent	Foils	Alkaline
Pleat	Quasi	Interpretation	
Plait	Permanent		
Interpretation			

Contraindications

Are there any contraindications which would limit a service or prevent a service from being carried out?

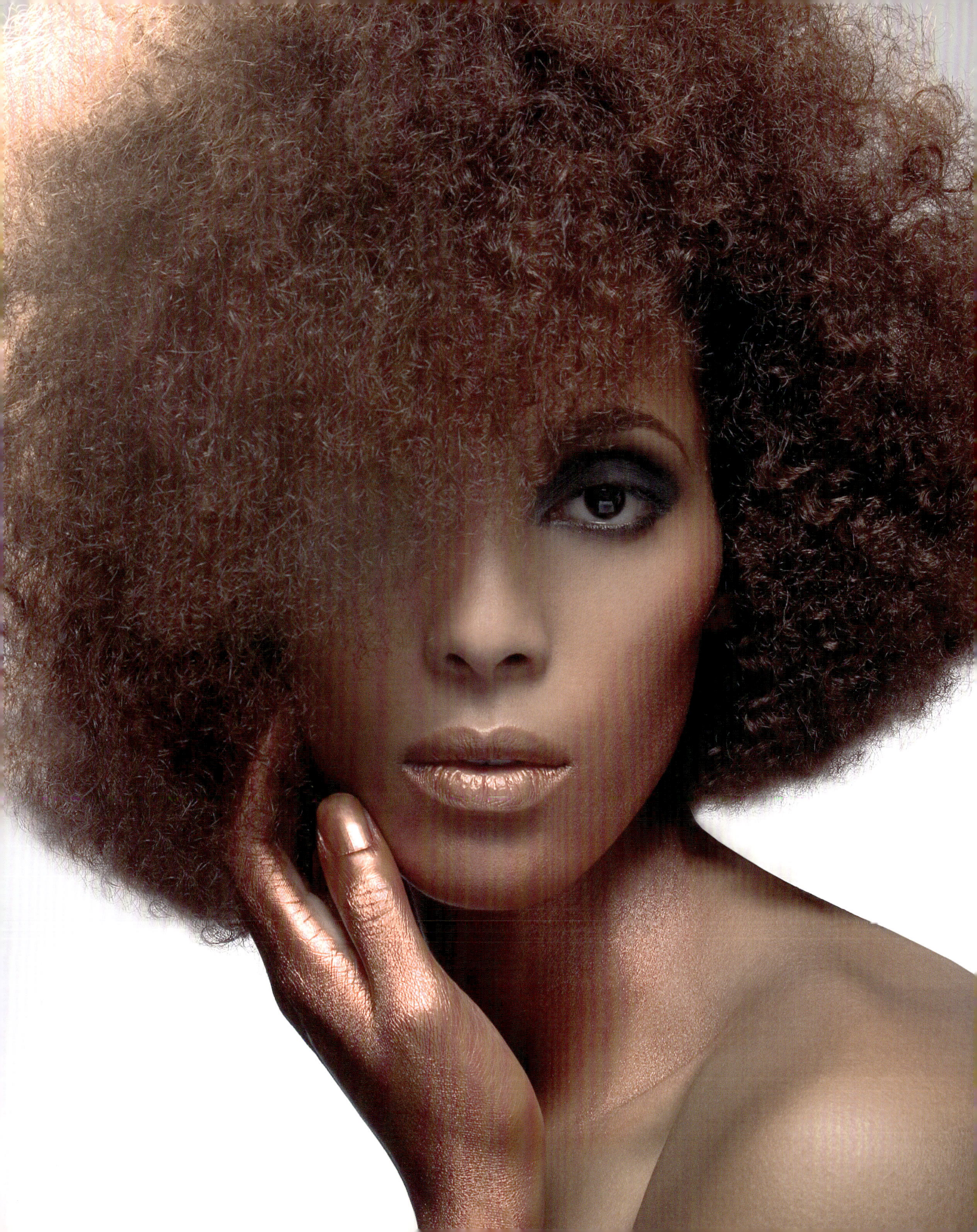

Style & Finish

Styling Techniques

Technique	Why used	When used
Roller set	To create movement, body, volume and curl on straight hair or to smooth and soften hair.	On wet hair
Velcro set	To create soft movement and body in hair; can be used while blow drying to create extra lift and movement.	On dry hair
Heated roller set	To create soft curl, wave, volume and body in hair; may be used prior to dressing hair into various shapes.	On dry hair
Pin curl set	Can be used to create very tight or soft curls, with or without root lift.	On wet hair
Finger waving	Used to create a waved look in the hair.	On wet hair
Blow dry	To give smoothness or movement and lift where required, power dry for speed. A variety of brushes can be used to create different effects.	Wet to dry
Tongs	To achieve curls of various degrees from soft waves to ringlets.	On dry hair
Straightening irons	Used to straighten and smooth the cuticle and prevent frizz, can also be used to introduce movement into hair. Gives an incredible straight finish.	On dry hair

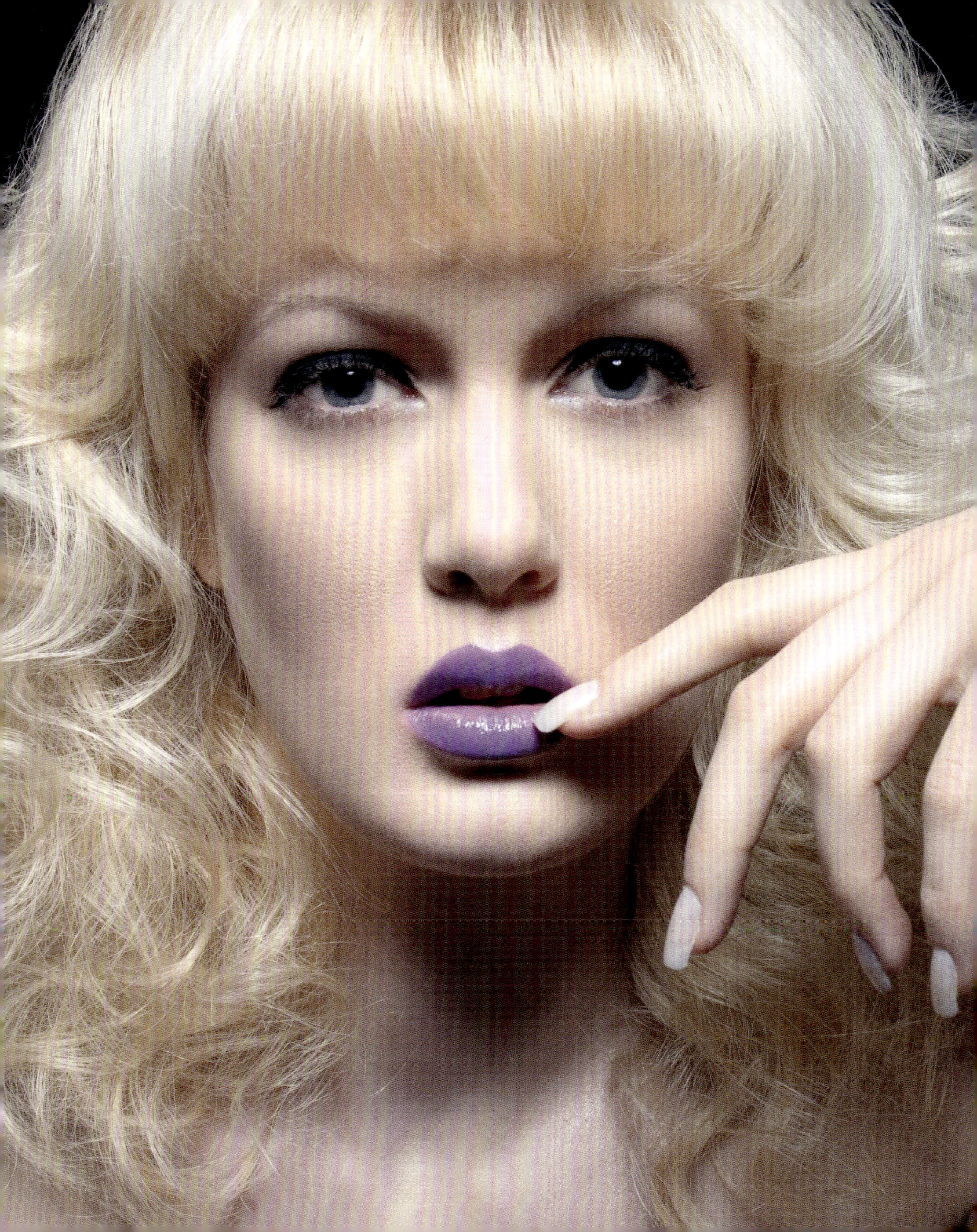

Blow Drying and Setting Theory

Hair is made up of polypeptide chains that twist together to form a shaft of hair as seen earlier. These chains are held together by disulphide bonds, weak salt bonds which help to hold the chains together and weak hydrogen bonds that prevent the loops of the polypeptide chain spirals from being stretched too far.

When hair is in its normal state it is not stretched. This state is known as the alpha keratin state. When the hair is stretched, as during the setting or blow drying process, it becomes beta keratin.

When the hair is wet and/or heated it is easier to stretch and will stretch further than when it is dry. This is because the hydrogen bonds and some of the salt bonds are broken by the moisture or the heat, so the springs (the shape of the polypeptide chains) can be lengthened.

When hair is set or blow dried it is stretched slightly by the rollers, fingers or by the brush. Because it is dried into this stretched position the broken hydrogen and salt bonds reform in a different pattern, and will stay there until the hair becomes wet or hot again. This is what gives a set or blow dry lasting power.

Hair becomes wet again by:

- absorbing atmospheric moisture
- shampooing
- being in a steamy bathroom or sauna
- excessive scalp perspiration
- being caught in the rain
- being in a humid climate

When the hair becomes wet or hot the hydrogen and salt bonds will go back to their normal pattern and the blow dry or set will be lost.

We must be aware of the dangers involved in the use of heated styling tools and equipment in the salon. If care is not taken there could be a risk of damaging the cuticle, causing the hair to break or burning the scalp.

As heat as well as water causes the hydrogen and salt bonds to break, hair should be held under tension until it cools down. It's not always necessary to hold the hair for a time while it cools, simply switch the dryer to a cool setting.

If heated equipment, such as tongs, are being used, avoid disturbing the hair until it cools. There are two main reasons why hair should be allowed to cool before finishing and dressing: to achieve a longer lasting effect, and to allow the hydrogen bonds to harden into their new position.

Depending on the desired effect and/or finish of the blow dry or set, it is essential to use the correct products on the client's hair. There is a huge choice in the ranges of products that are available for use when drying, setting and finishing hair. The most frequently used styling/setting products are: lotions, mousse, activators and gel. The most frequently used finishing products are: dressing creams, sprays, and wax. The products used in the salon are also available as retail products.

Tools for drying, setting, styling and finishing hair include a range of combs and brushes designed to achieve various effects. The choice of tool used often depends on the length of the hair, the type of hair, the texture of the hair, the density of the hair and the amount of volume and movement required – in addition to your own and your client's personal preference.

As fashions and trends in hairdressing change, techniques used to achieve the look also change. The most common techniques used for styling hair are: blow drying, power drying, finger drying, and setting techniques that include the use of rollers, pins, tongs and heated electrical equipment.

Before choosing a technique, take into consideration the following factors:

the required result

the haircut

the texture and elasticity of the hair

the length and density of the hair

the growth pattern around crown and hairline

the head and face shape

The Haircut
This will affect the choice of style that can be achieved.

The Texture and Elasticity
Hair that is over-processed will have reduced elasticity and may not curl as well as hair with good elasticity. Hair that is very strong may be difficult to style and require more tension when setting and drying.

Hair Growth Patterns
The client may have difficult or strong hair growth that will determine the direction of the look.

Hair Length and Density
The hair may be too short or too long for a specific style. Density: the hair may be too sparse or too abundant for a look or for a particular technique.

Head and Face Shape
The choice of the style must complement the head and face shape of the client.

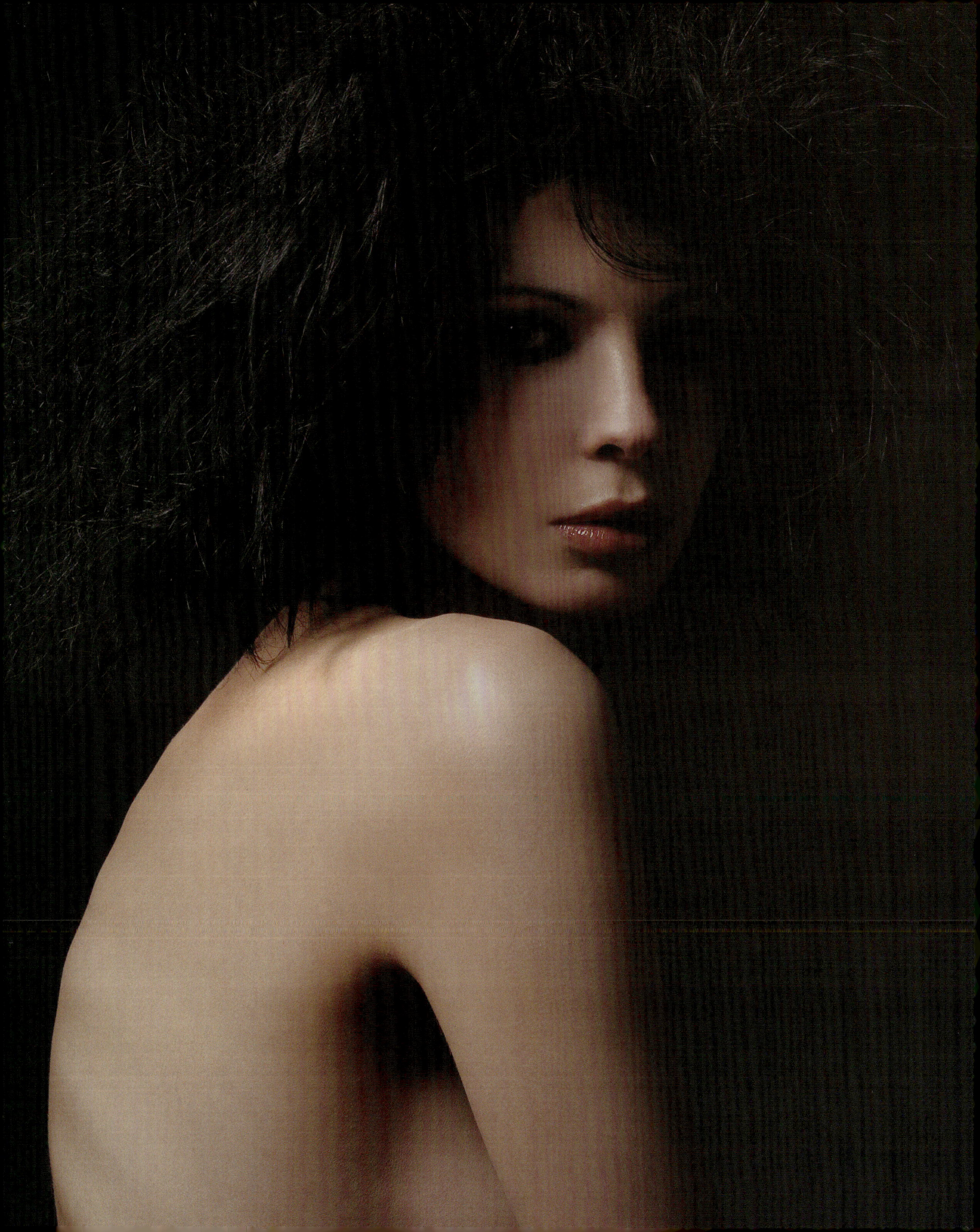

Developing Technique

At this stage, we have covered a variety of skills which include the significance of choosing the correct equipment to work with. We have analysed hair and skin structure and learnt the importance of client hair care. By now you will have a better understanding of client consultation and how to advise clients correctly. You have progressed with blow drying skills by using a variety of brushes to create various finishes. Setting on wet or dry hair has come in to focus, with an exploration of basic methods and sectioning patterns. Next we will examine the Technique Cuts Collection which demonstrates eight basic cutting techniques for women and then moves on to barbering for men, taking you through three haircuts. The chapter on barbering also guides you through scissor-over-comb and clipper work techniques. The remaining chapters of the book demonstrate techniques in colour, permanent wave and finally, hair up. You will be perfecting your skills as you explore the universal world of hairdressing, and building your confidence as you progress. Strive to develop and achieve excellence by practising and refining your skills.

The *Technique* hairdressing educational programme fuses motivation, ideas and creativity. The highest standards of technical expertise and innovative training have been combined to provide a forward-thinking approach to today's hairdressing. Training is the key to personal development and it is through continuous training and dedication that each individual can progress to the highest level in modern hairdressing.

Through continual development over time, hairdressing techniques have evolved. A thorough understanding of these techniques can be mastered to give you the knowledge on which all commercial, advanced, and fashion techniques are based. *Technique* now moves to a further examination of the methods that will enable you to create hairstyles that are fashionable, classic and adaptable.

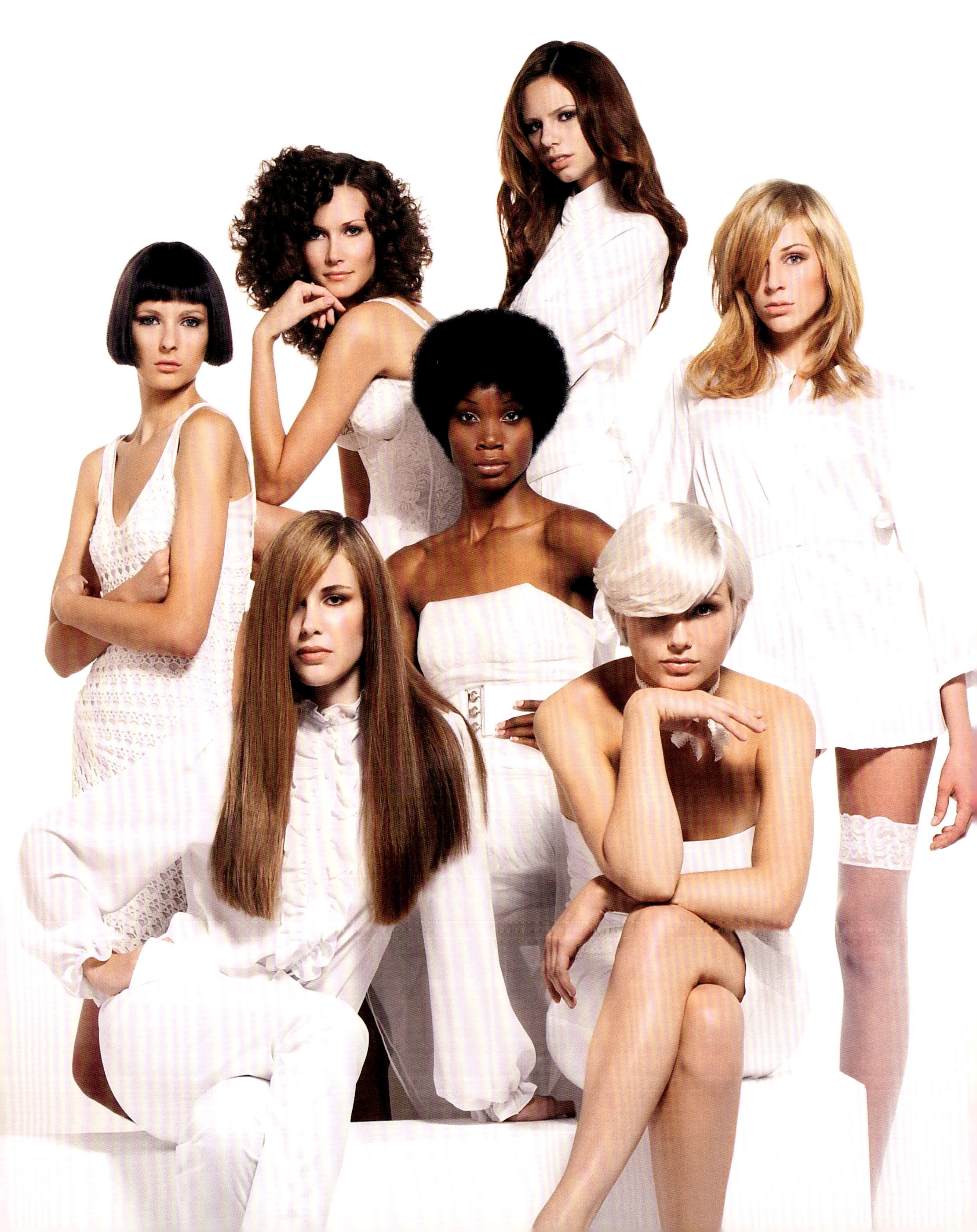

Technique Cuts Collection

Technique Cuts is a collection of haircuts which will give you the technical basis for all commercial, fashion and advanced techniques. A true understanding of the Technique Cuts Collection is the key to further progression.

Once mastered, the basic principles of the Technique Cuts Collection will strengthen and enhance any previously gained expertise.

As trends and fashions change, this collection of haircuts allows for these changes. It is important that we adapt hairstyles to our clients, reflecting their face, personality and lifestyle. When working with these techniques, a variety of shapes can be created, simplified or adapted to suit each individual client. This will enable you to produce work that is fashionable, commercial and adaptable while maintaining a high standard of technical expertise and a progressive approach to your work.

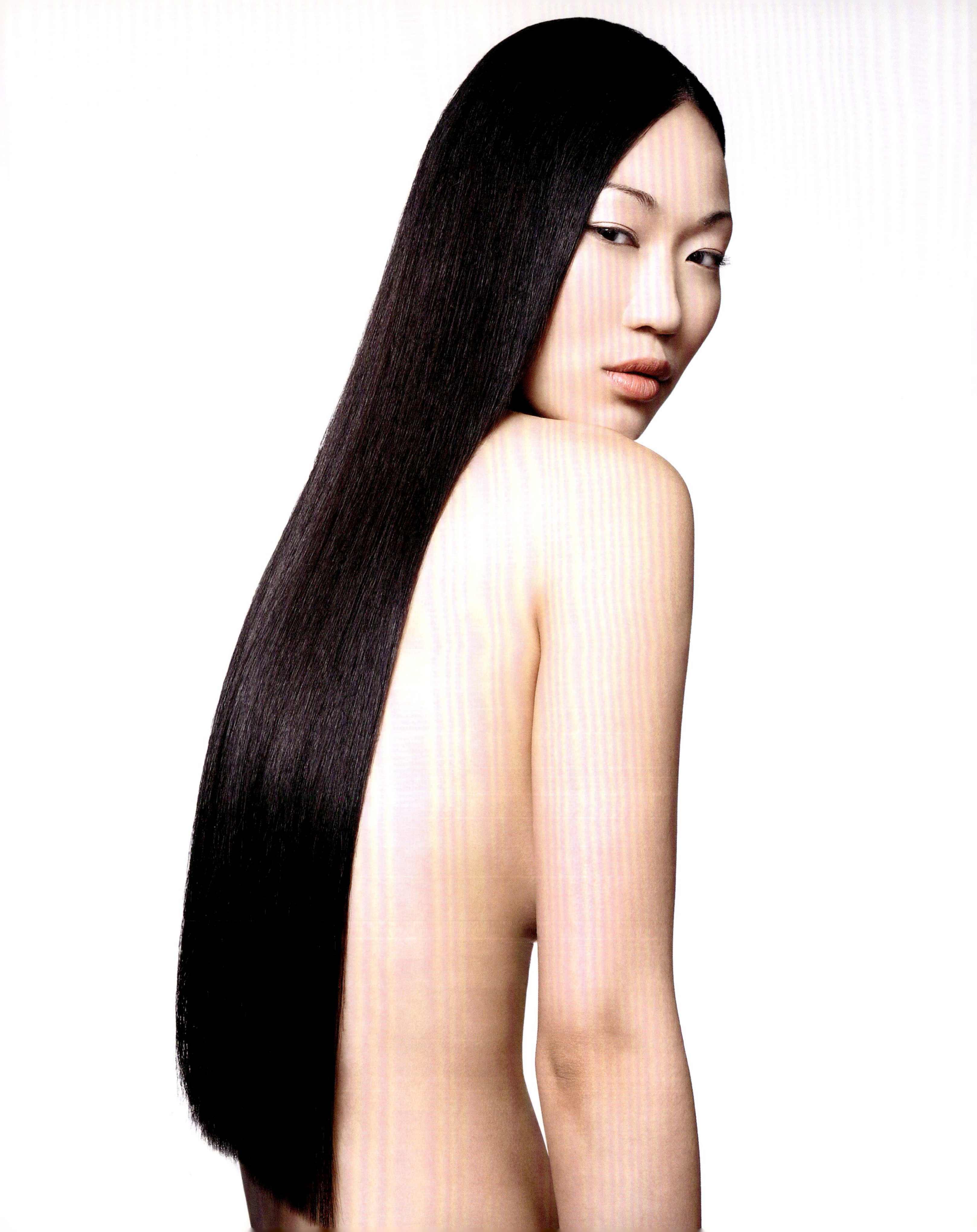

The One Length Cut

When cutting a guideline, it is essential that the balance remains consistent, especially in the case of a precision haircut. The one length cut is an ideal shape as a first haircut for the apprentice hairdresser. This cut introduces the hairdresser to reference points of the head, guidelines, section patterns and terminology. The one length cut falls below the shoulder and includes an over-directed technique which increases length towards the front, framing the face. This cut is perfect for the client who wants to maintain a longer style, with a very simple shape created by working all the hair to a one-level perimeter.

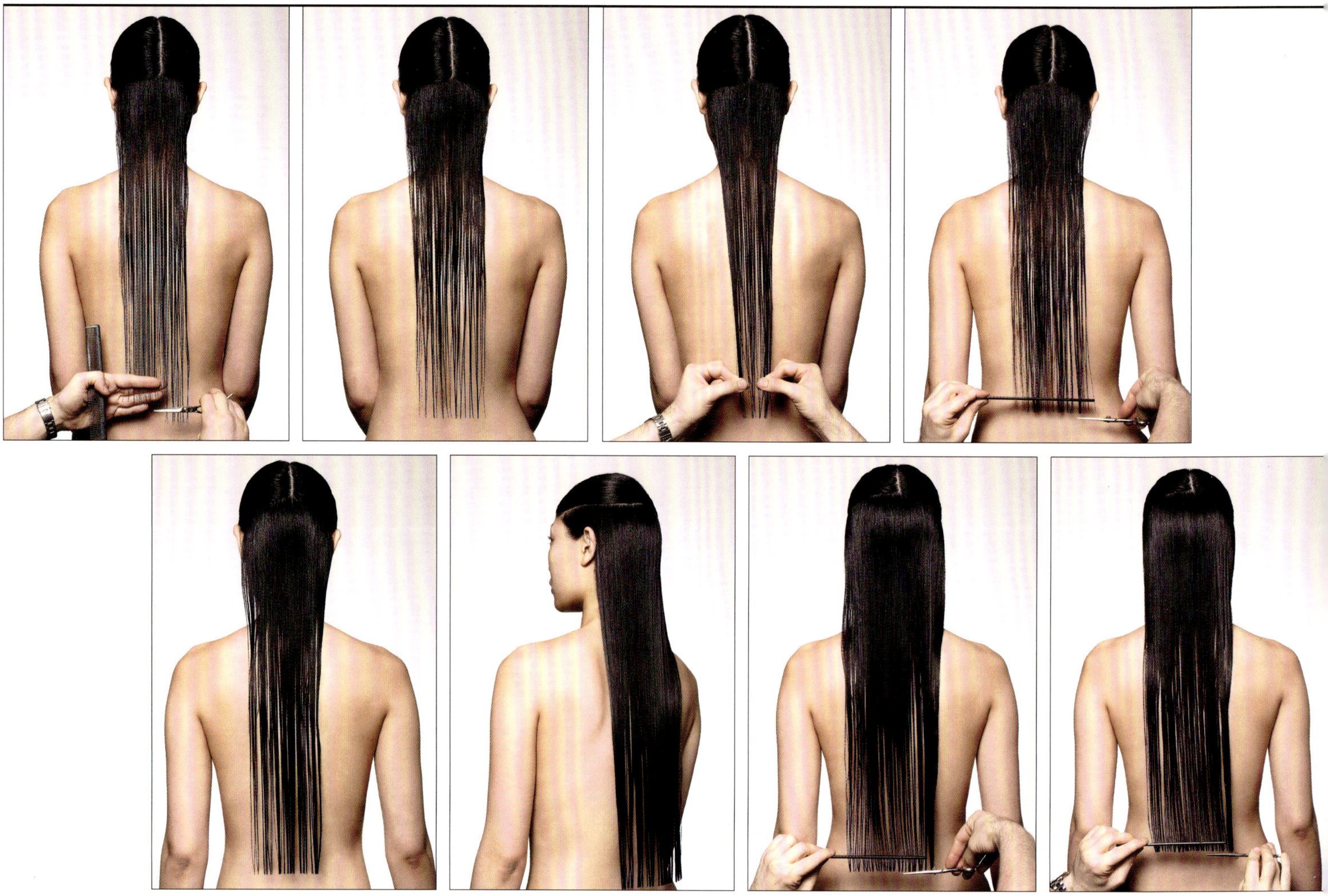

1 For the cut, after shampooing and conditioning, the hair is parted with a central division, from forehead to nape. This parting is called a profile line.

2 With the head in an upright position, from the centre back, two horizontal sections are taken, about 3cm deep, depending on the thickness and texture of the hair. This section will form the baseline for the cut. Starting at the centre back, comb the hair cleanly downward, holding between the fingers with maximum tension.

3 Combing the hair down to its natural fall, a line is cut across the back of the shoulders. Cutting the hair cleanly and squarely across, from the middle at the centre back out to each side.

4 The balance is checked by pulling the outer edges into the centre back. The line must balance correctly as this baseline is the guide for all proceeding sections.

5 The next sections are taken working up the back of the head. Take horizontal sections on both sides of the head; combing the hair down to its natural fall, cut the hair using the baseline as a guide.

6 As you progress to the occipital bone, take a horseshoe section at the centre back on the occipital bone to the recession area on both sides of the head.

7 Over-direct the side and front sections, by working them around the ears into the baseline at the back of the haircut, and cut using the guide line.

8 Continue up horizontally to the profile line, and over-direct the side, front and top sections towards the back and continue cutting a square line across the back of the shoulders.

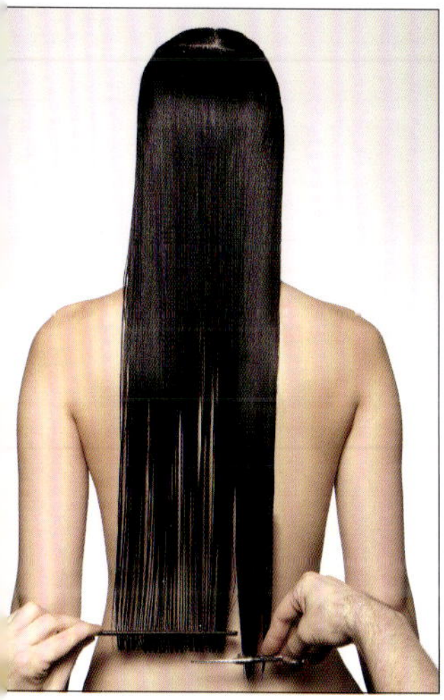

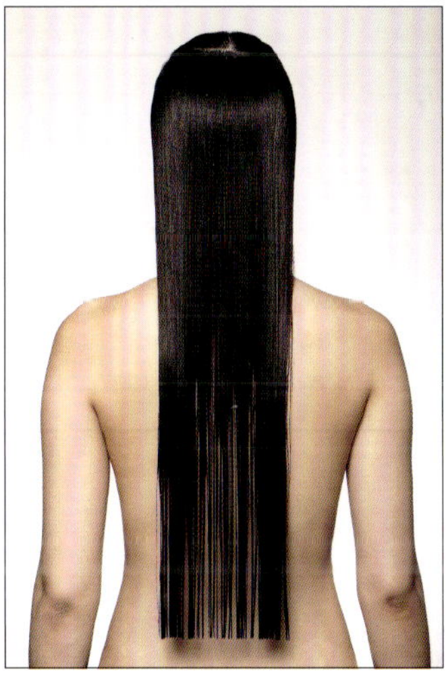

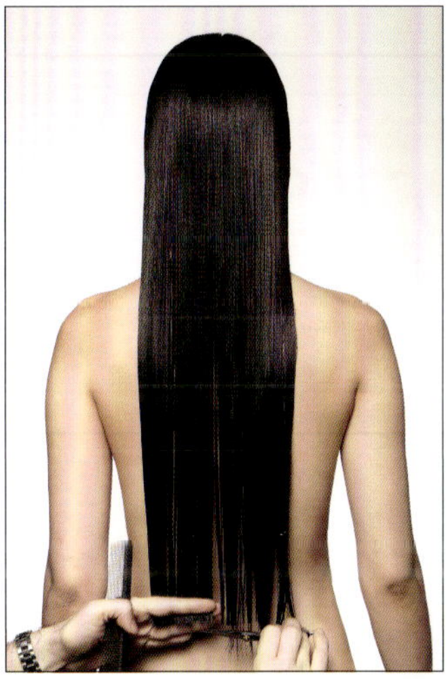

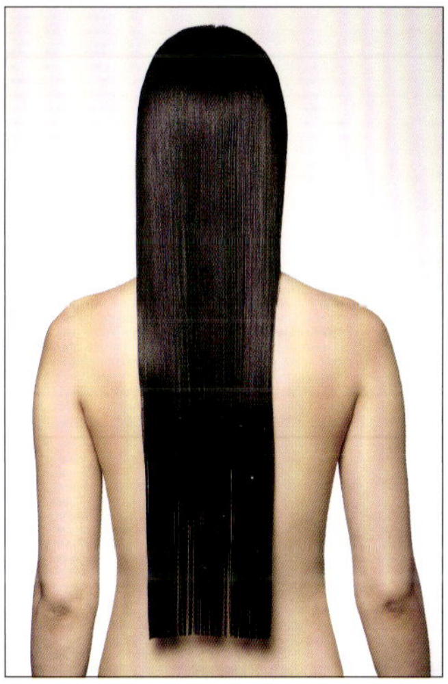

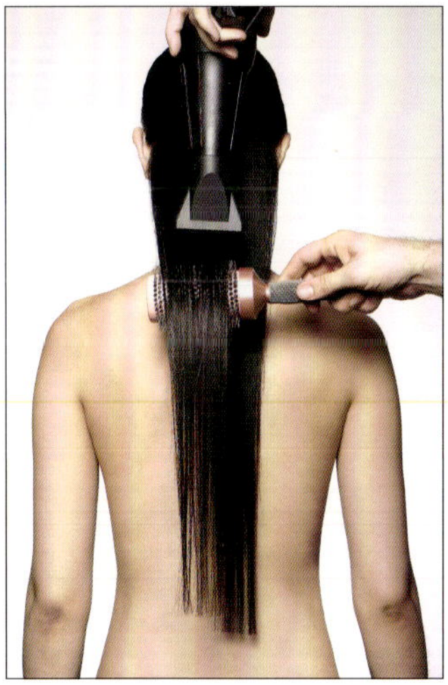

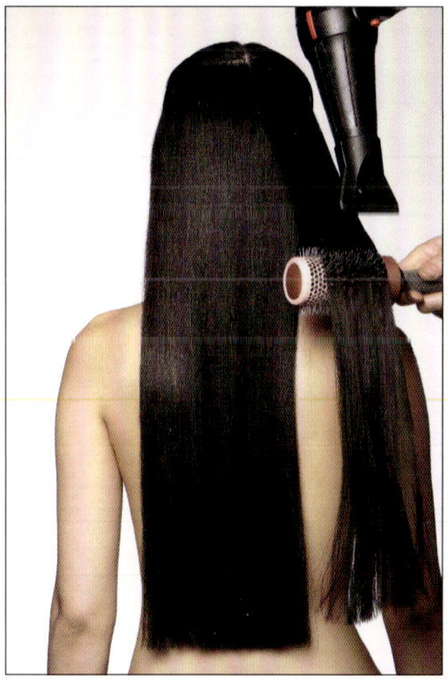

9 The balance on both sides of the head is checked by pulling the back, side and front sections into the centre back.

10 The one length haircut is complete.

11 For the finish, use an appropriate styling product and distribute through the hair evenly.

12 To create a smooth, straight finish the hair is blow dried using a nozzle on the hairdryer; use a large metallic round brush – this will achieve maximum smoothness on the hair and create shine.

13 The hair is dried using the same sectioning pattern as used for the haircut. Direct the hairdryer downward onto the hair and keep a good tension on the hair for a straight smooth finish. Dry the hair using the same sectioning pattern as in the haircut.

14 Apply a finishing product to the hair, such as hair glaze or shine mist, a finishing product will promote a smooth finish and healthy shine to the hair.

15 By bending the client's head forward you will see some graduation, simply cut away any graduation which may have built up during the initial cut.

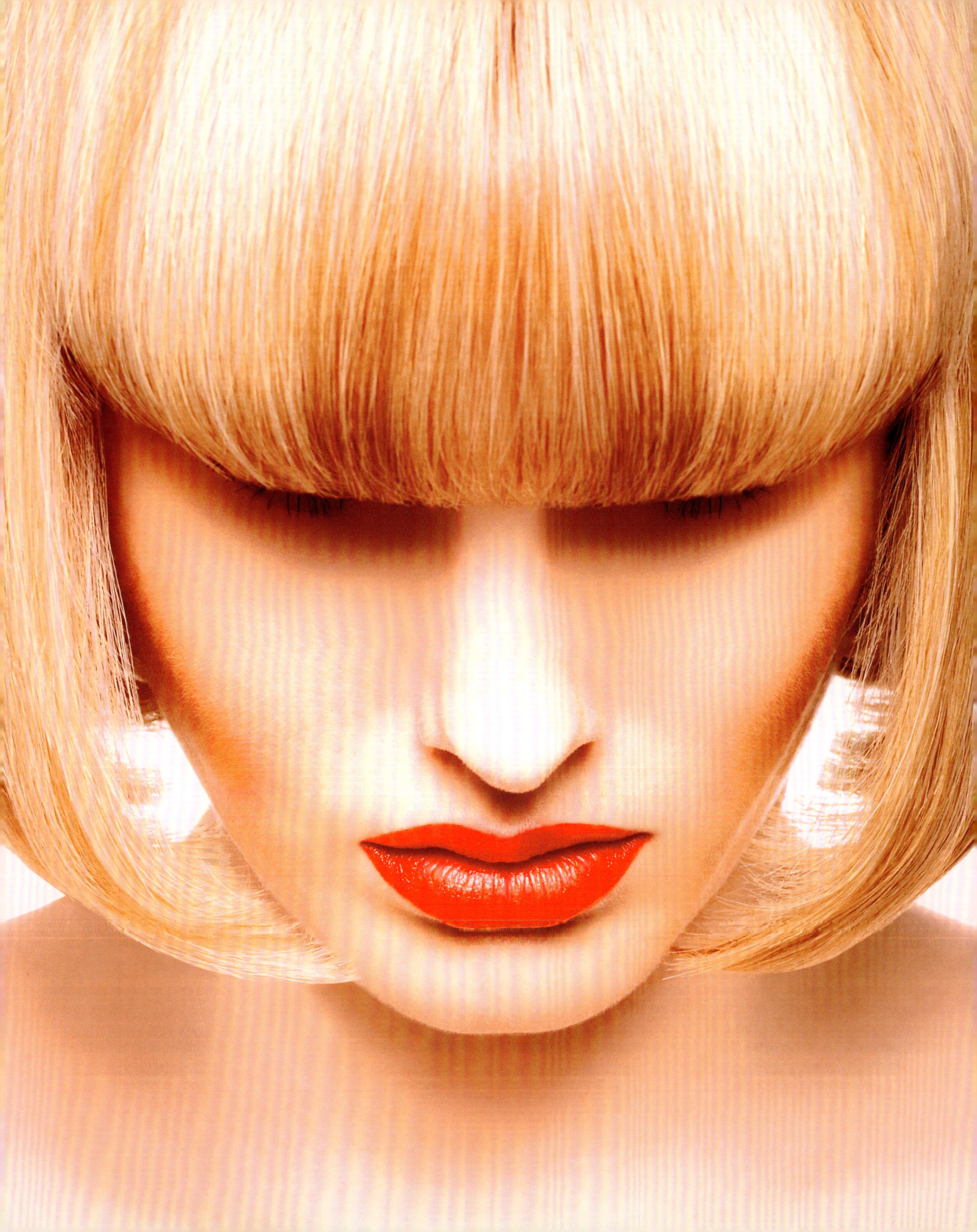

The Classic Bob

This timeless classic shape can be worn in a variety of ways with many variations. The classic bob is suited to most textures and face shapes.

Essentially the classic bob is a one length shape, above the shoulders with or without a fringe. The fringe, if worn, is a focal point of the cut. Proportions of the cut and of the client's face should be taken into account when deciding on the length of the bob. The classic bob is a precision cut which can be blow dried smooth with the ends turned under, or alternatively, maximising the bluntness of the cut, it may be ironed straight to emphasise its natural swing. The bob was considered to be the sign of a liberated woman when first worn in the 1900s.

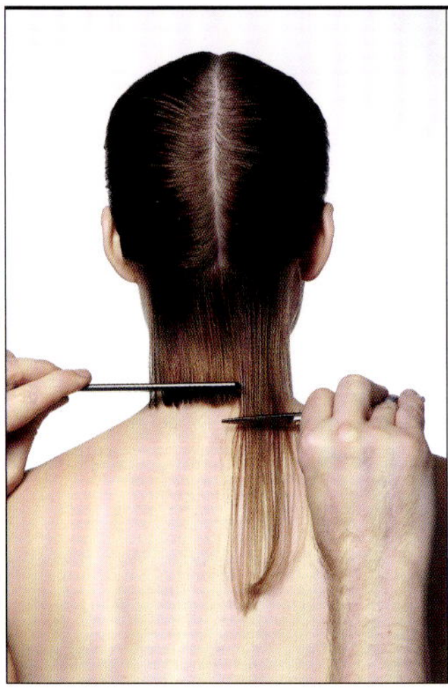
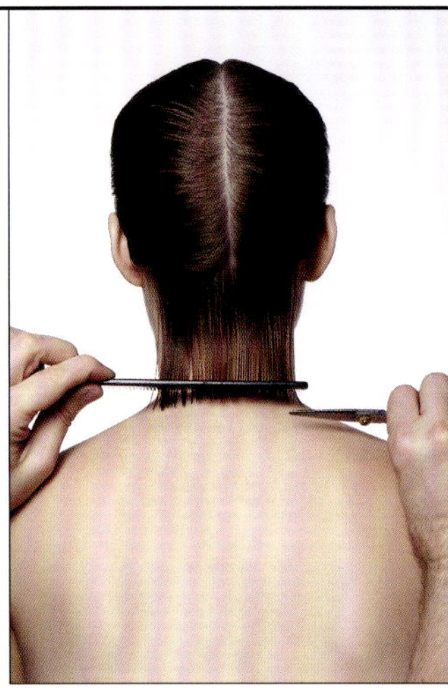
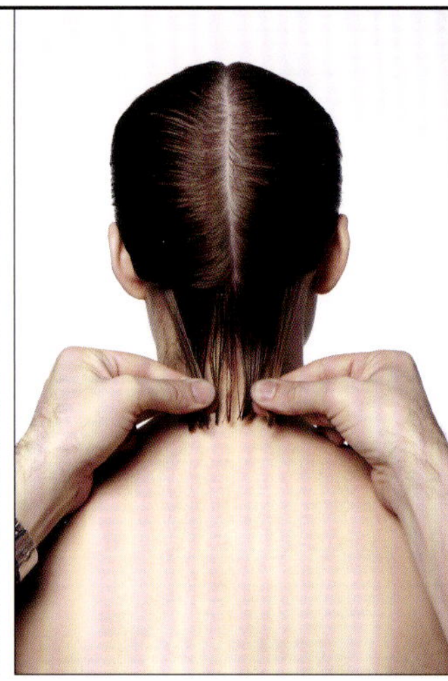
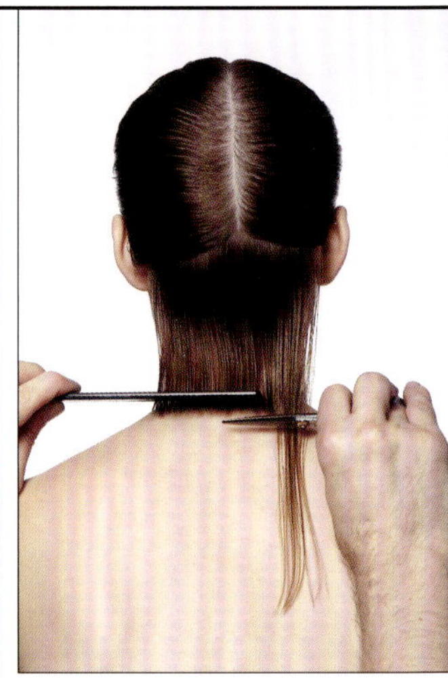

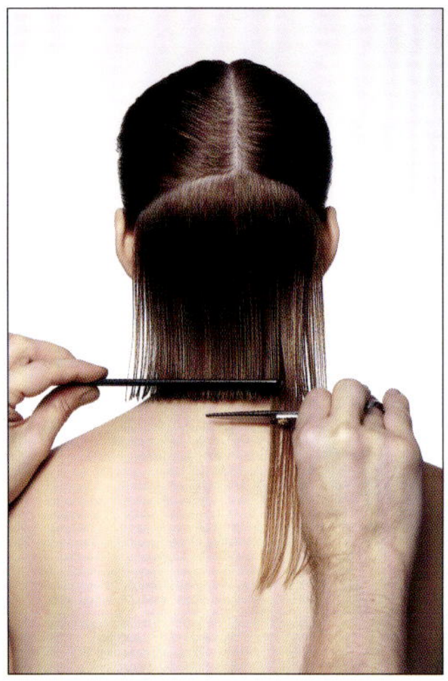
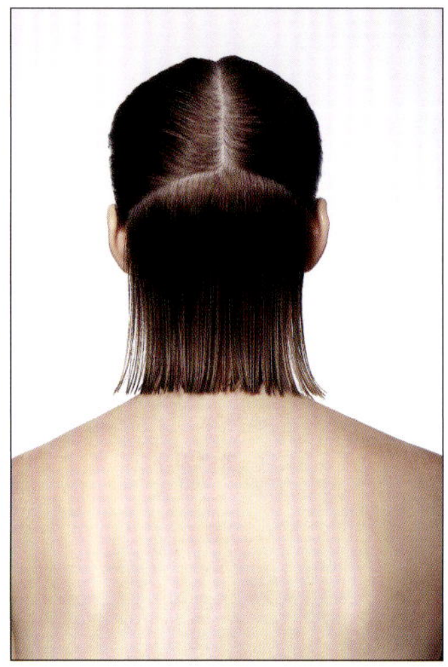
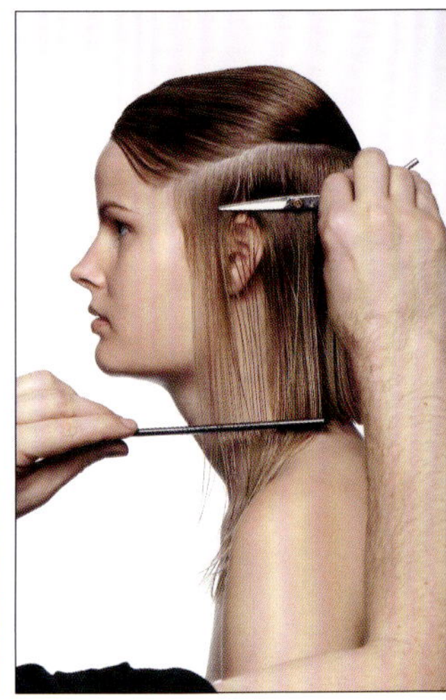

1 For the cut, after shampooing and conditioning, the hair is parted centrally using a profile line from forehead to nape.

2 With the head in an upright position, two horizontal sections are taken at the nape about 3cm deep – this depends on the thickness and texture of the hair.

3 The hair is combed down to its natural fall; with minimum tension this section is held in place with the comb, the baseline is cut squarely across the nape from centre back to the outer edges on both sides of the head. By cutting just underneath the comb this technique creates a very straight line, which forms the basis of the classic bob.

4 With the guideline in place, check the balance by pulling both outer edges into the centre back. If level move on and progress.

5 Continue up the back of the head taking horizontal sections, each section is combed down to its natural fall and held in place with the comb. The underneath guide line is then followed.

6 At the occipital bone, take a horseshoe section and comb the hair down to its natural fall. Start at the centre back and work around to the sides; at this point pay attention to the ears: allow them to protrude through the section. With the hair held in the comb continue cutting the line squarely across.

7 The same line is cut on the other side of the head and the balance is then checked before continuing.

8 Horizontal sections are taken up both sides of the head and combed down to a natural fall from the profile line. Each section is held in the comb and the guide line followed. The balance is then checked again, on both sides of the head.

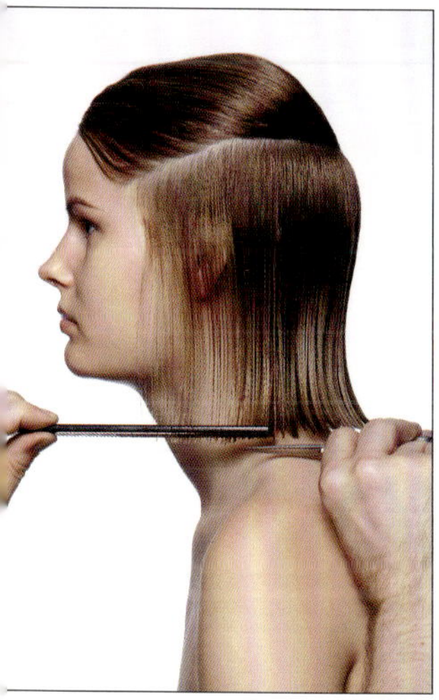
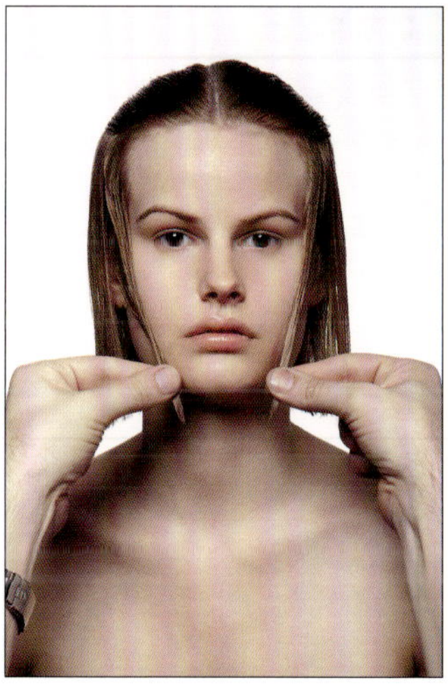
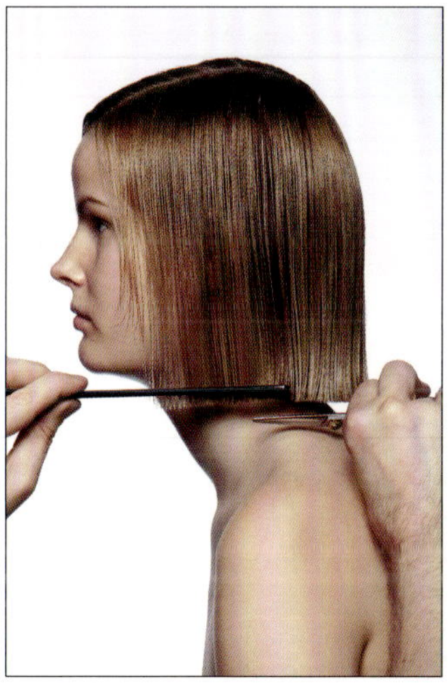
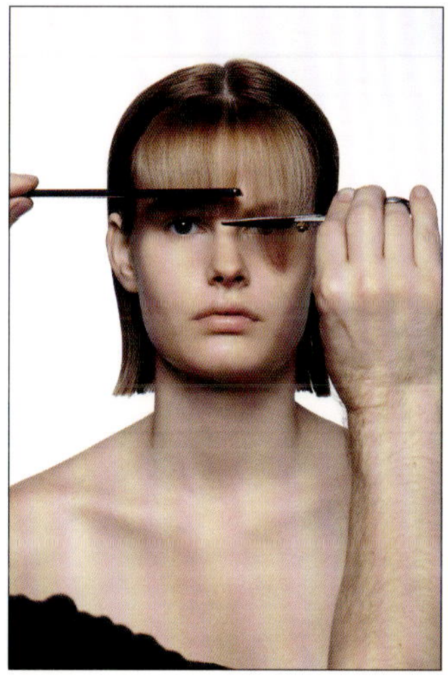
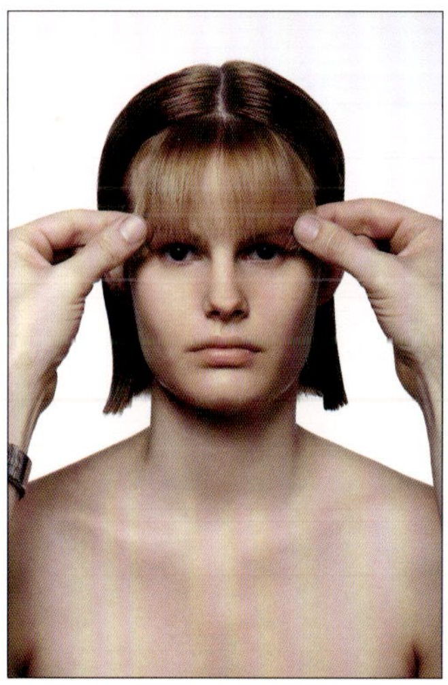
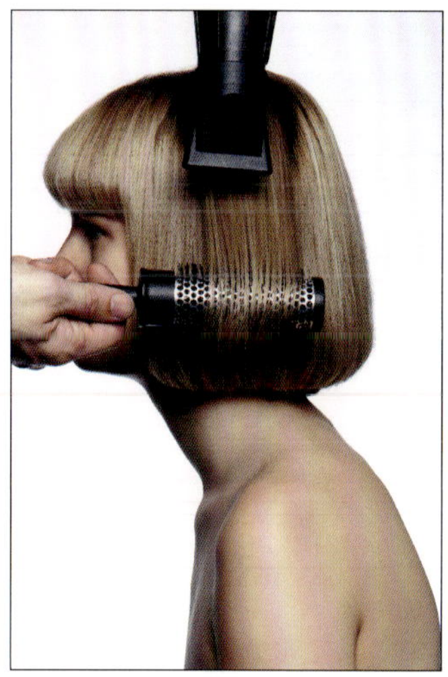

9 The fringe can be cut damp or dry. Cutting a fringe dry will allow for natural root lift and accuracy of the desired length will be achieved.

10 The fringe area is separated by using a V-shaped section which is taken from each recession area and across the profile line.

11 The length of the fringe is determined by the eyebrows and is also a personal choice. When cutting a fringe it is advisable to not extend the fringe beyond the ends of the eyebrows, unless fashion and face shape dictate.

12 For the finish, use an appropriate styling product and distribute through the hair evenly.

13 To create a smooth and shiny finish, blow dry using a Denman brush and use a nozzle on the hairdryer. Keep a good tension on the hair while drying the hair straight.

14 Starting in the nape area, dry the hair using the same section pattern as was used in the cut, direct the hairdryer downward onto the hair to create a smooth and shiny finish.

15 Apply a finishing product to the hair, to promote shine. Check the haircut after drying.

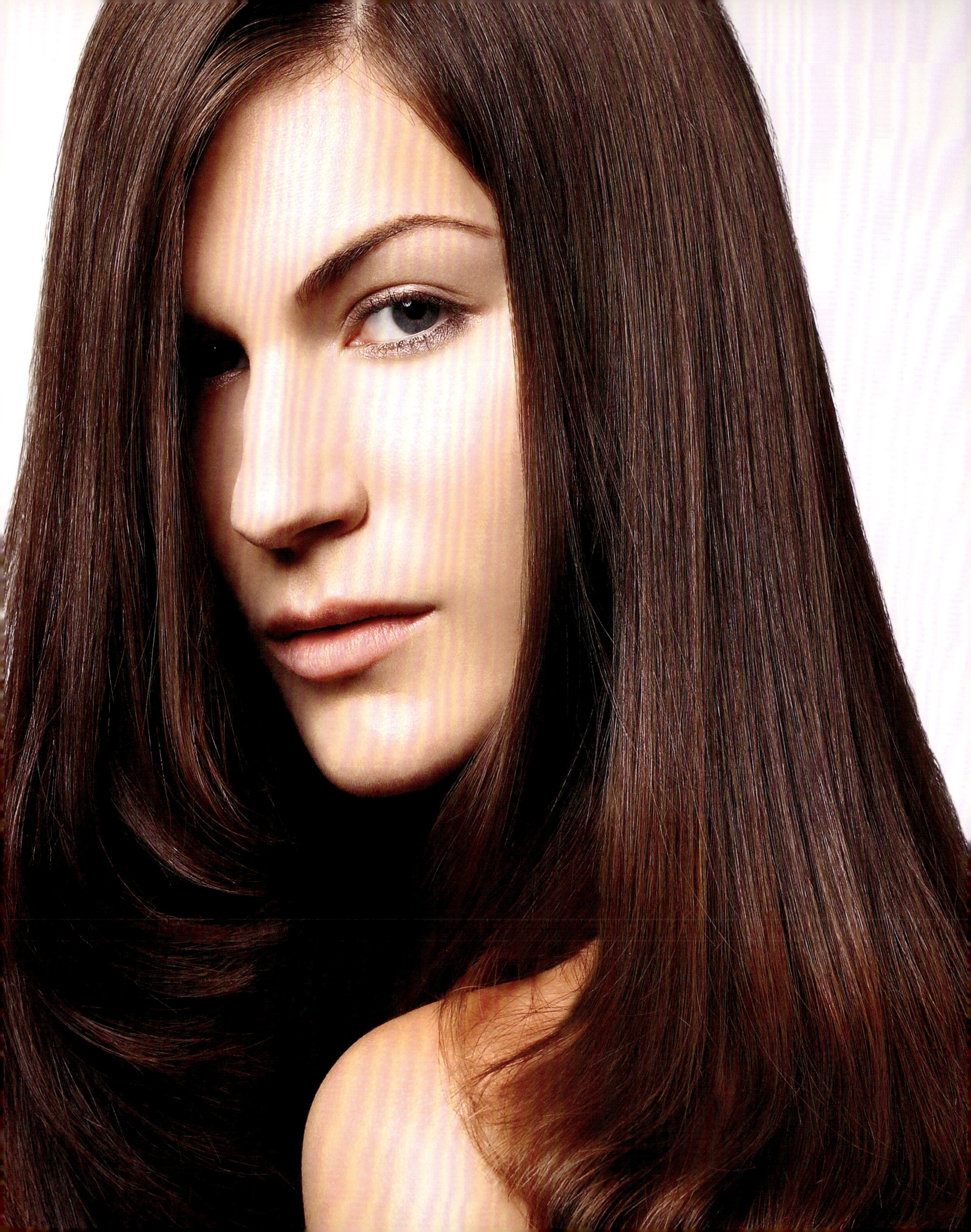

Forward Graduation

Forward graduation works through exactly the same technique as that of the one length cut. Progressing from the baseline, take a diagonal back section and decide upon the length the graduation will take – again take into account suitability and proportion. This angled graduated line can bring out the client's natural features as this shape frames the face. Forward graduation is a one length cut which falls below the shoulder; it's a very versatile shape. The graduation around the face can be left as a solid graduated line, or it could be pointed into with the scissors for softness and texture; this would depend on the natural texture and density of your client's hair.

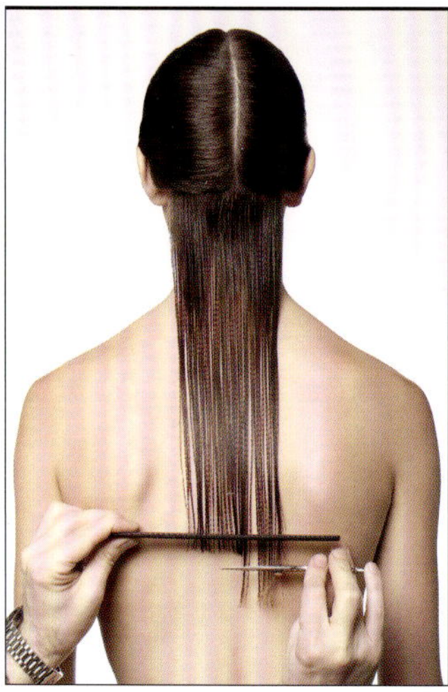
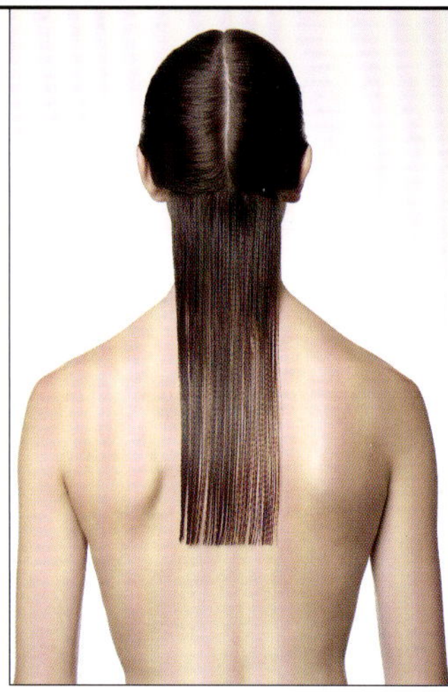
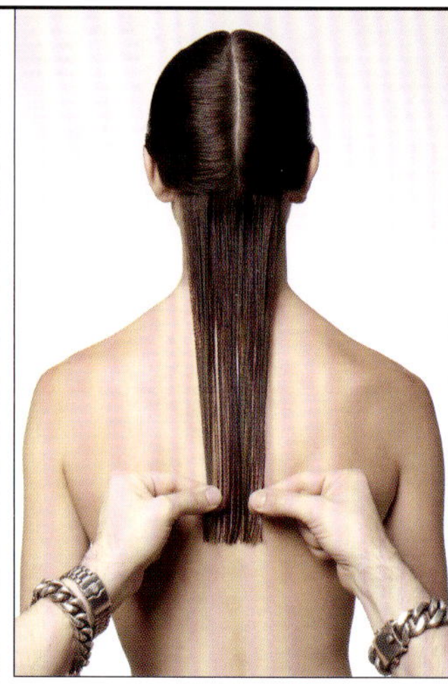

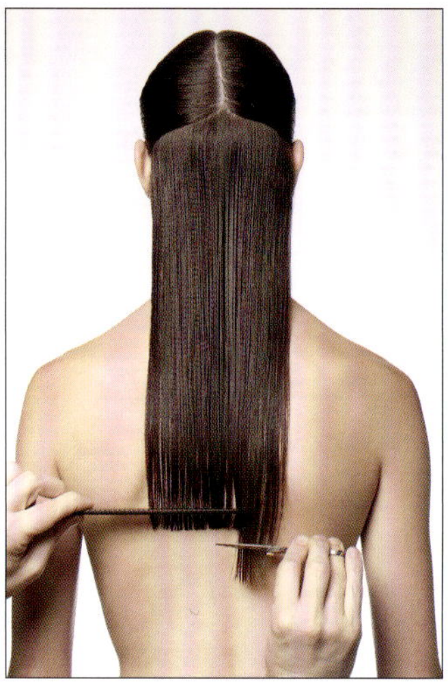
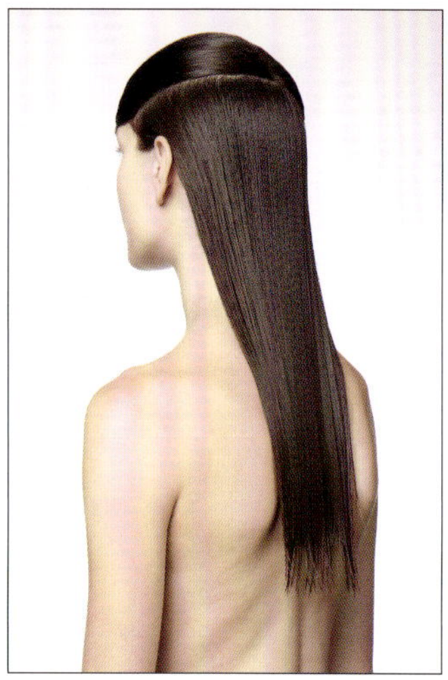
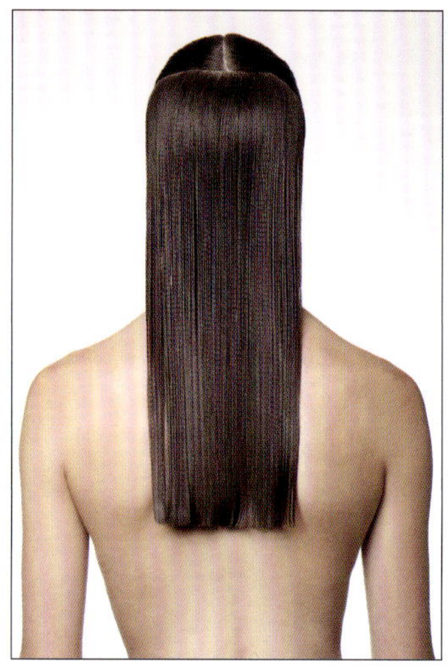
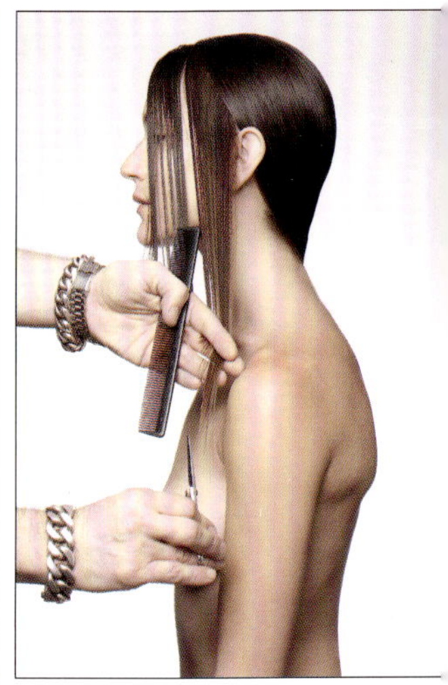

1 For the cut, after shampooing and conditioning, the hair is parted centrally using a profile line from forehead to nape.

2 With the head in an upright position, two horizontal sections are taken at the nape about 3cm deep – this depends on the thickness and texture of the hair.

3 The hair is combed down to its natural fall. Working either through the fingers or the comb, the base line is determined. Cut the base line from the middle at centre back out to each side. Check the balance by pulling the outer edges into the centre back.

4 Progress up the back of the head with horizontal sections, each section approximately 3cm deep, combing the hair down to its natural fall. Cut the hair, following the base line as a guide, cleanly and squarely across the back of the shoulders in a straight line.

5 At the occipital bone take a horseshoe section into the recession area on both sides of the head. Over-direct the side and front sections into the baseline at the back of the head, cut and follow the guide. Work in horizontal sections up to the profile line; then, when all the sections have been cut, check the balance.

6 From the front, at the profile line, take a diagonal back section to the apex of the ear about 3cm in from the hairline. Work equal distribution on both sides of the head.

7 Combing these sections down to their natural fall, a line is cut visually, up from the baseline to nose, lip or chin level. The level at the front depends on the client's preference or the length of hair that is being worked with, as a fringe may already be incorporated within the haircut.

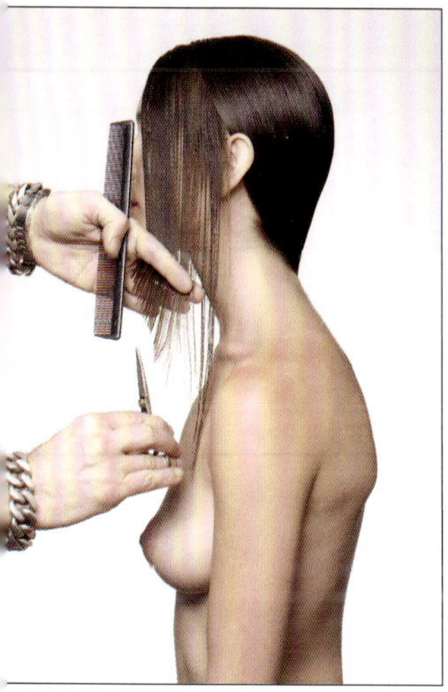

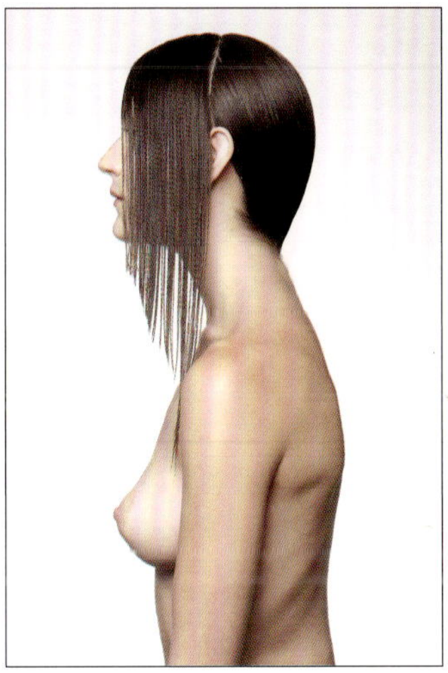

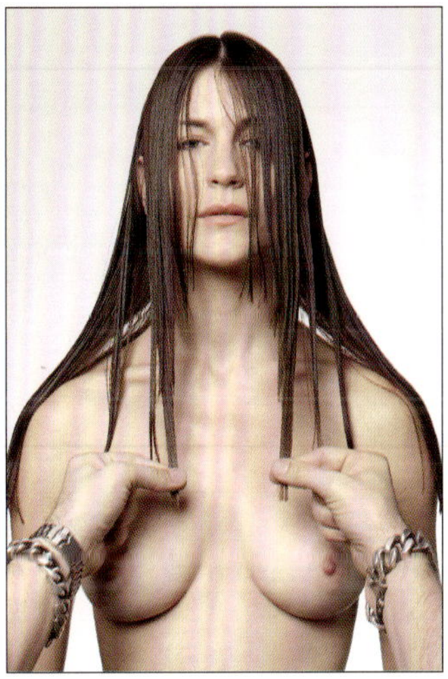

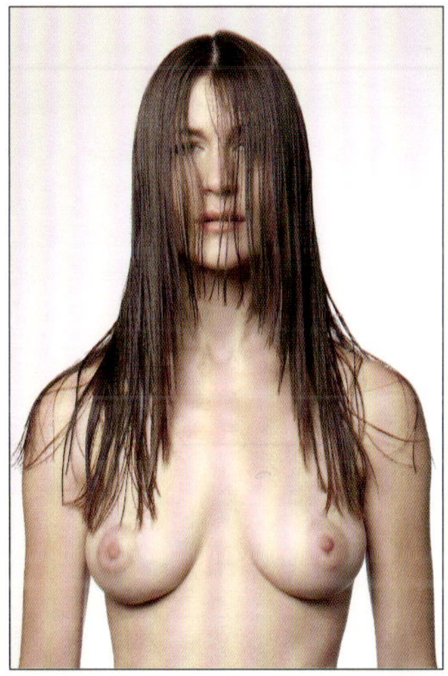

8 Cut exactly the same line on the other side of the head and then check the balance by pulling fine sections of hair from key areas on the head into the centre front, cross-checking the balance at the front and working down to the baseline.

9 The next section is taken in a wedge, thicker at the profile line, finer at the apex. This section is combed down to its natural fall and cut following the guideline.

10 Continue working back to a radial section, when both side sections have been cut; from the profile line comb all the hair down to the natural fall and check the balance. The haircut is now complete.

11 For the finish, use an appropriate styling product and distribute through the hair evenly. To create a smooth, straight finish, blow dry the hair using a nozzle on the hairdryer. Use a large metallic round brush to achieve maximum smoothness on the hair to create shine.

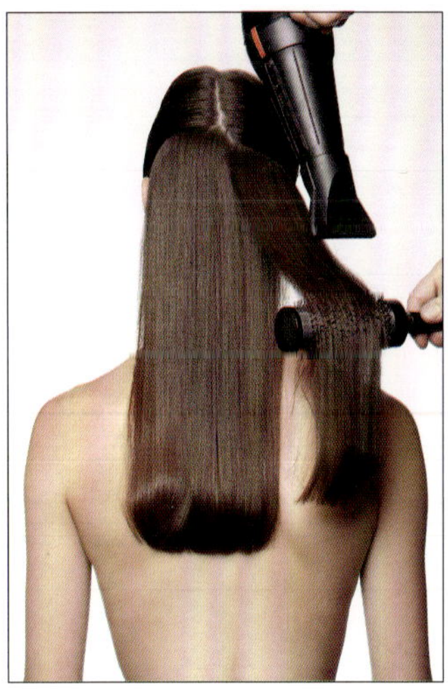

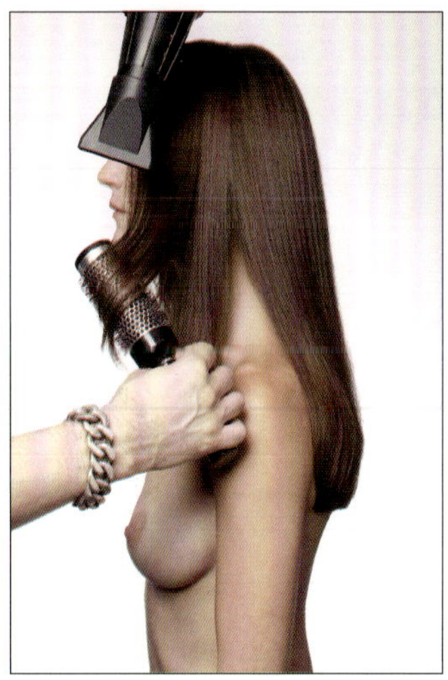

12 The hair is dried using the same sectioning pattern as used for the haircut. Direct the hairdryer downward onto the hair and keep a good tension on the hair for a straight smooth finish.

13 Check the haircut for any imperfections. Apply a finishing product to the hair, such as a hair glaze or shine mist. Applied onto the surface of the hair, finishing products promote a smooth finish and healthy shine to the hair.

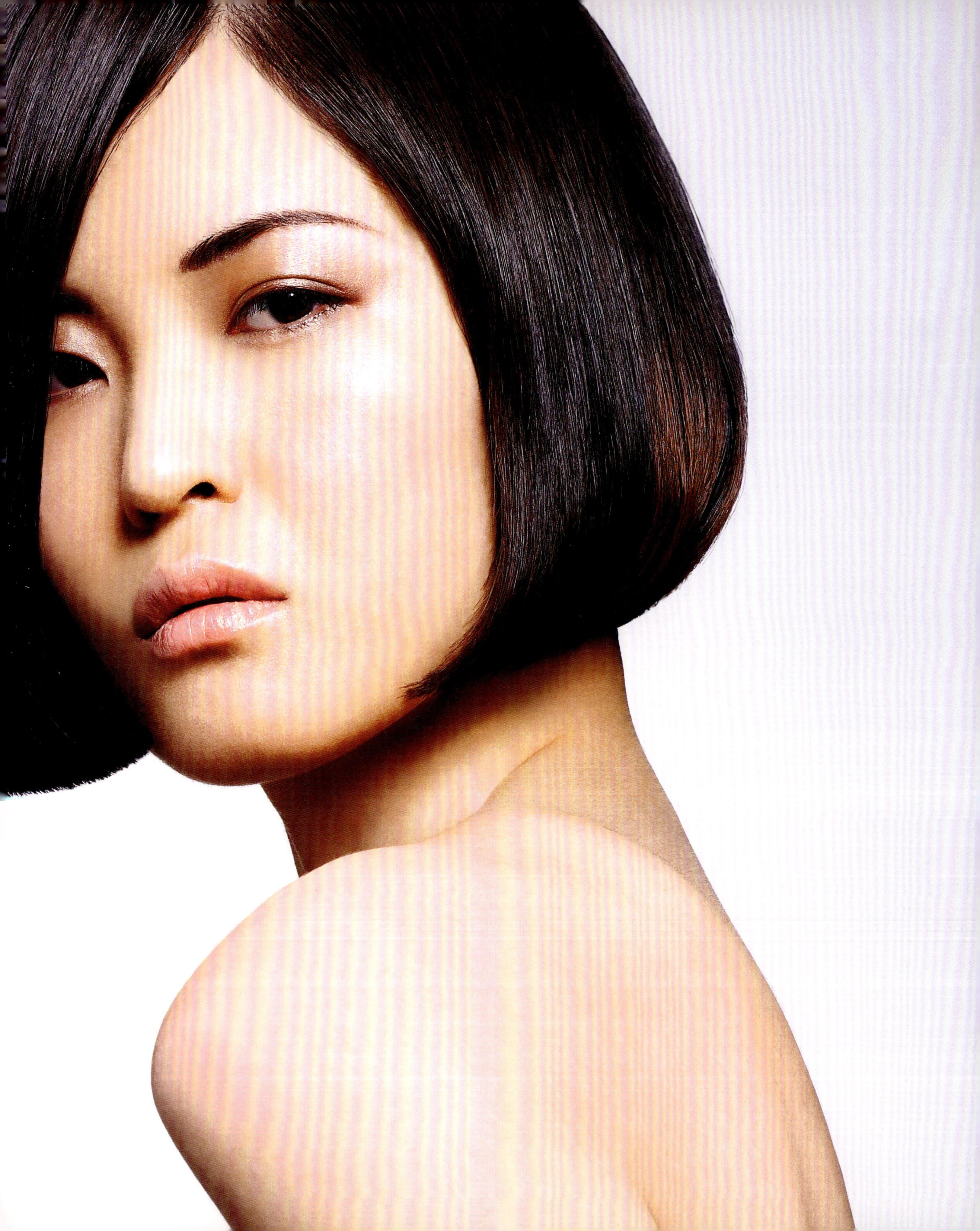

The Graduated Bob

The graduated bob is a variation of the classic bob. This haircut will give a very strong sharp silhouette. A graduation technique builds weight between the nape and occipital area, working into one length through the sides of the haircut. To successfully create this shape it is essential that you check that the client has a hairline that lies flat in the nape area. This is because the outline is cut relatively short and hugs the nape. The graduated bob is a geometric shape which is young and fun and really creates a strong statement. For maximum impact this shape is best worn without a fringe.

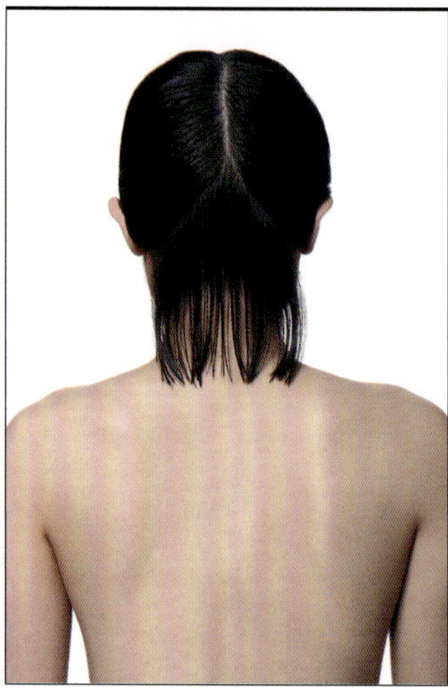

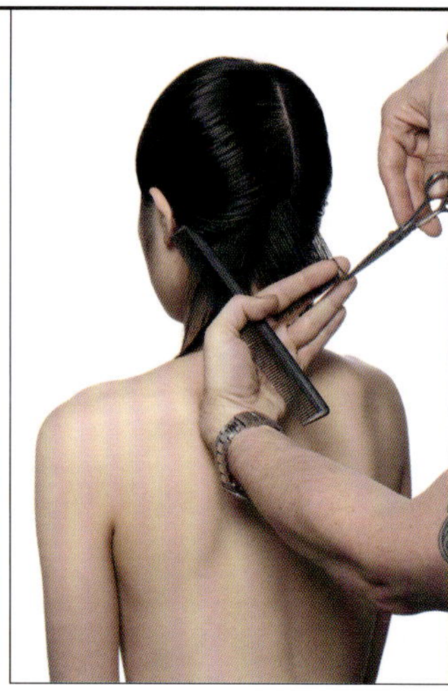

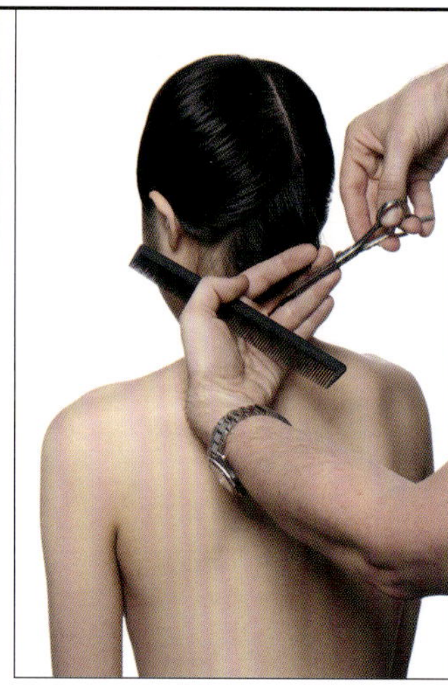

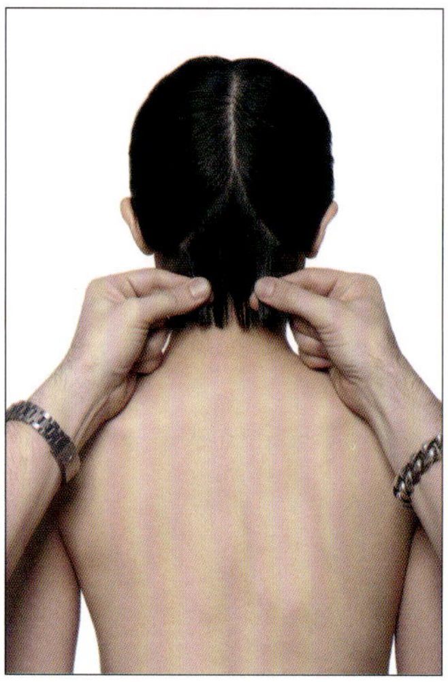

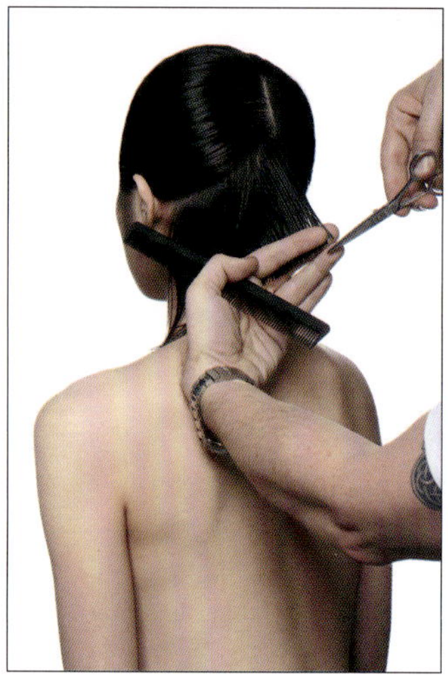

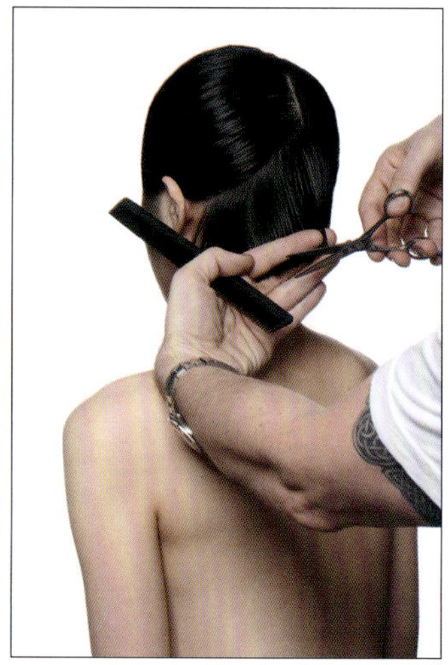

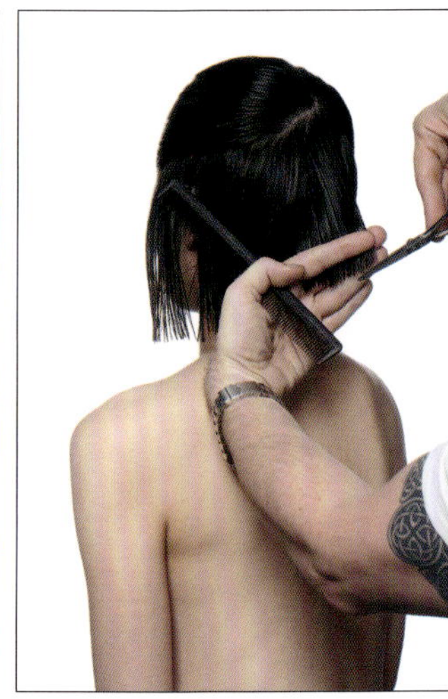

1 For the cut, after shampooing and conditioning, the hair is parted centrally using a profile line from forehead to nape.

2 With the head in an upright position, two diagonal forward sections are taken from the profile line to behind the centre of each ear.

3 From the centre back take subdivisional diagonal forward sections on either side of the profile line and pull out at 45 degrees. Then layer down the nape into the hairline.

4 Using the top of this section as a guide, a wedge-shaped section is taken from centre back out to the right hand side of the nape; pull this section out at 45 degrees and layer down into the hairline.

5 Continue working around this side of the nape into the hairline and follow the guideline. Pull out each section to the same level of graduation and layer down into the hairline.

6 The final section in the nape is pulled out parallel to the diagonal forward parting, and graduation continued.

7 Repeat exactly the same sectioning pattern on the left side of the nape, working in wedge-shaped sections at 45 degrees and layer down to the hairline.

8 Just above the occipital bone, two diagonal sections are taken from the profile line to behind the top of each ear.

9 In the centre of this section a sub-section is taken and held out to the underneath graduated guide line.

10 Wedge-shaped sections are taken and continued around the back of the head and, finishing parallel to the diagonal parting, each section is pulled out and down to the graduation guide line. Use the same sectioning pattern on the other side of the head.

11 The following sections at the back of the head are taken from the crown to the top of each ear. Comb down these sections and follow the graduation guide line underneath.

12 Connect the sides to the back by taking a diagonal forward section from the crown to the recession area, on both sides of the head. Comb this section down to the natural fall, allowing for the protrusion of the ear; working from the graduation guide line, continue the line to jaw level. Cut this line on both sides of the head. Check the balance on both sides of the haircut by pulling sections down from in front of each ear.

16 On completion of the blow dry, graduation at the back of the haircut is then cross-checked for weight distribution and any excess heaviness is removed by picking up sections in the comb and point cutting into the hair to remove weight.

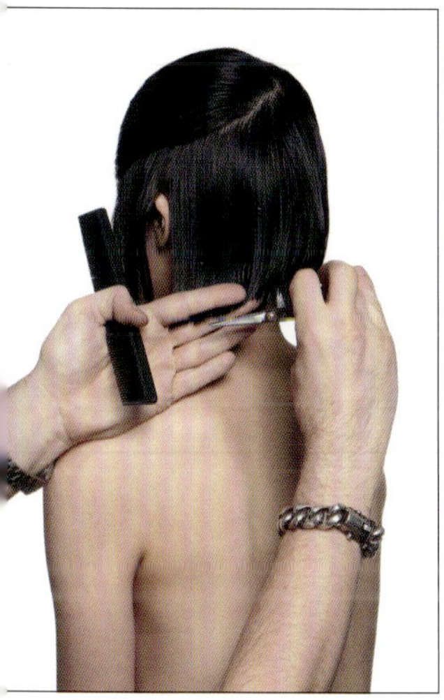
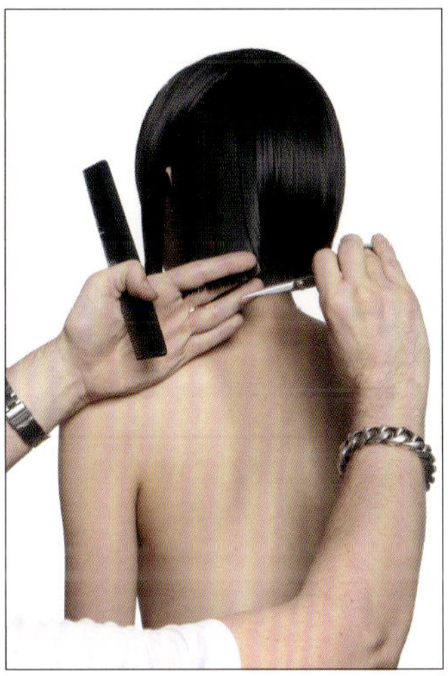
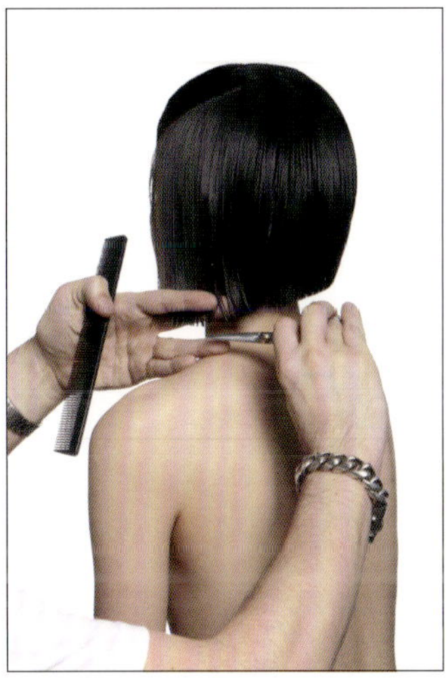

13 Take the following sections horizontally from the crown to the top of the recession area; comb down to the natural fall and use the base line as a guide. Continue working up the head to the profile line, slightly over-directing the front sections into the base line at the sides of the haircut. Repeat this exact same procedure on the other side of the head.

14 The balance of the haircut is then cross-checked on both sides.

15 For the finish, use appropriate styling product and distribute evenly through the hair. To create a smooth finish, start at the nape and use a Denman brush. The hair is blow dried flat in the nape then, working up the back of the head, follow the same sectioning pattern as used in the haircut, turning the ends under throughout the blow dry. Direct the air flow from the hairdryer downward onto the hair, smoothing the cuticle and creating a glossy finish to the hair.

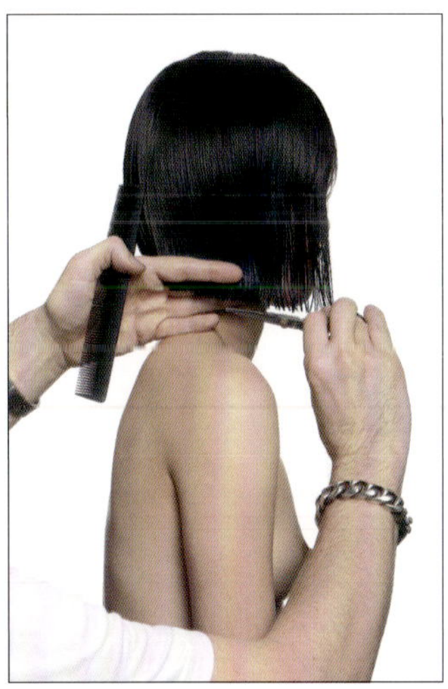
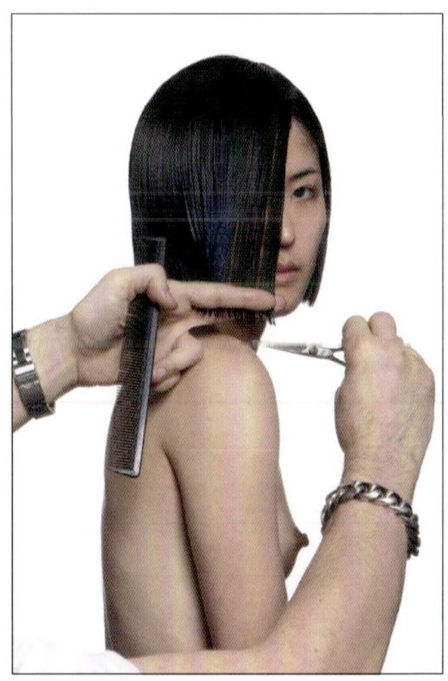

17 The parameter in the nape area will need either softening or strengthening for more definition; personalise this area to complete the graduated bob.

18 Apply a finishing product to the hair, such as hair glaze or shine mist. Applied on to the surface of the hair a finishing product will promote a glossy shine to hair.

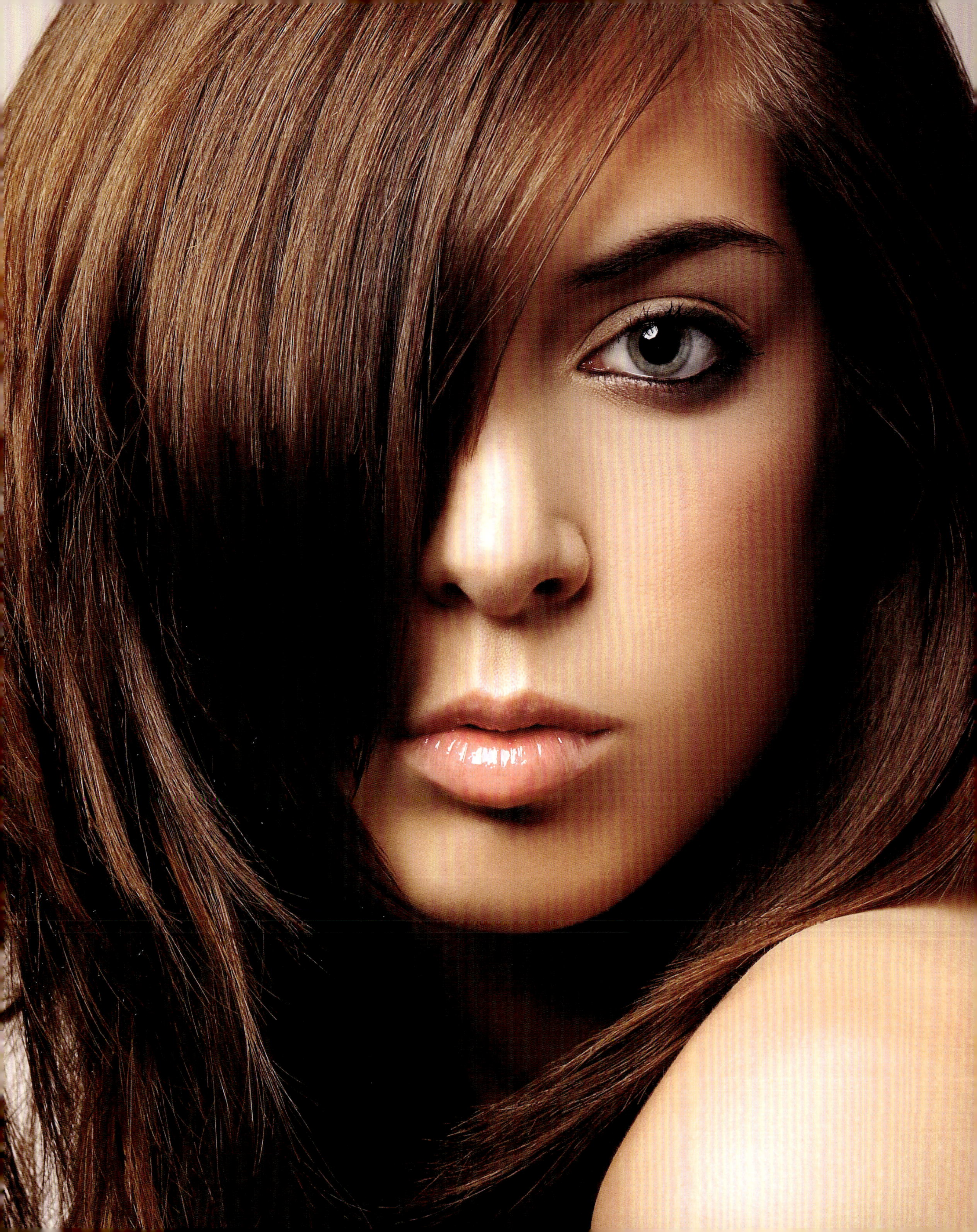

Square Layers

The square layer haircut is a truly versatile shape which can be cut below the shoulder or sit directly on the shoulder line. Square layers haircut works through both the one length and forward graduation techniques. The layers will create movement and softness within the shape while maintaining a degree of weight towards the baseline. A fringe of varying lengths can be incorporated and worked by sweeping across the face, this will add softness and femininity; again, think about proportion on both perimeter and internal layering. When the hair is dry, further texture can be achieved by slicing into the hair – this will shatter the shape and give seamless layering.

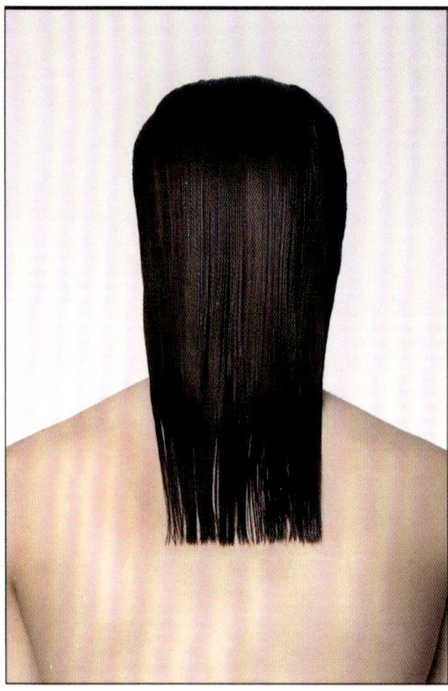

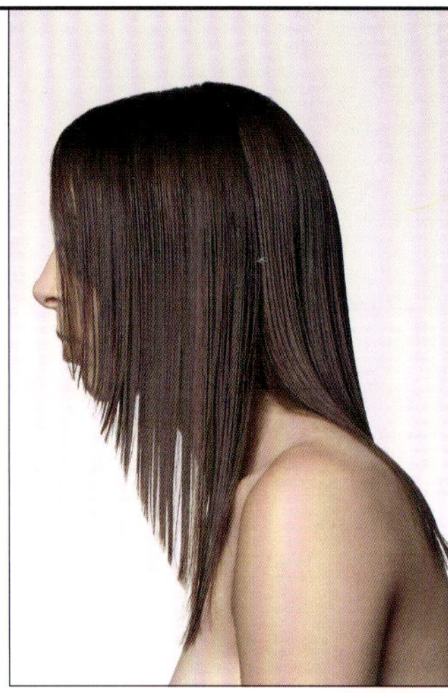

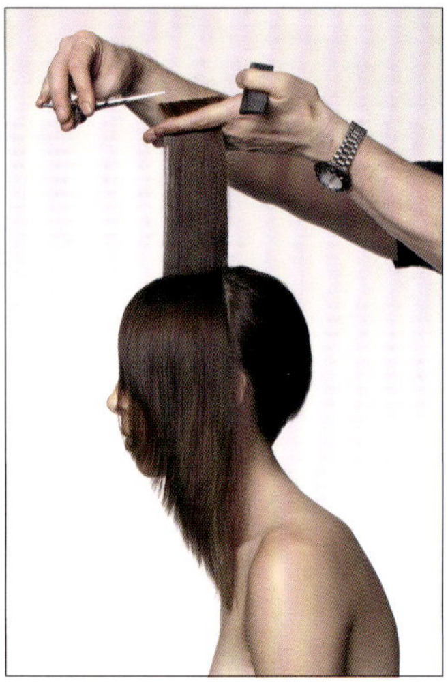

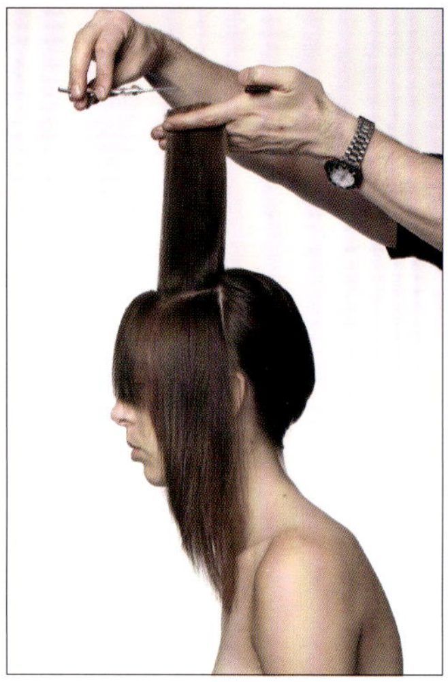

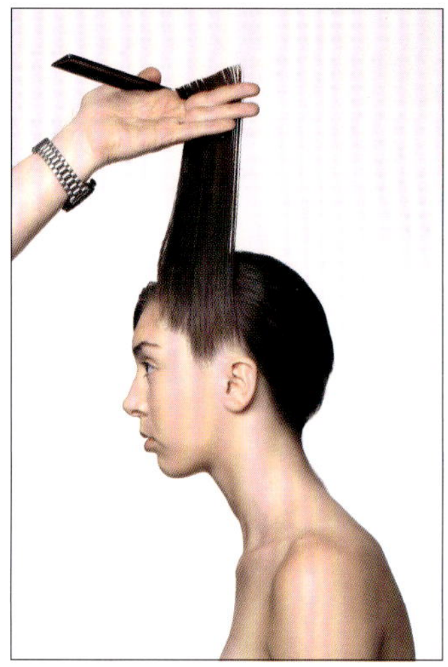

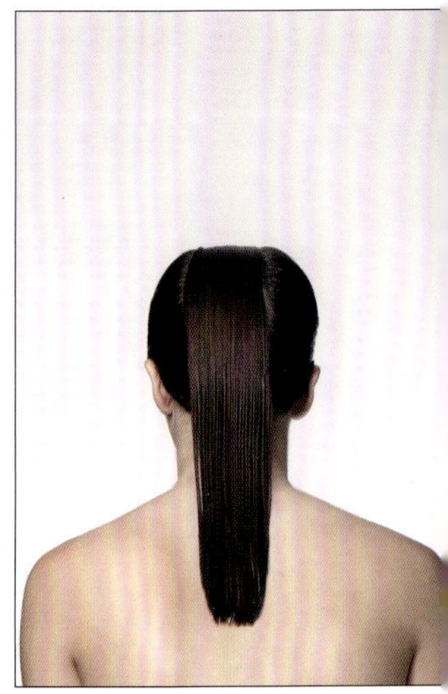

1 For the cut, after shampooing and conditioning, the hair is parted centrally using a profile line from centre forehead to centre nape.

2 With the head in an upright position, two horizontal sections are taken at the nape about 3cm deep – this will depend on the thickness and texture of the hair.

3 The hair is combed down to its natural fall. Working either through the fingers or the comb, the base line is determined. Cut the baseline from the middle at centre back out to each side. Check the balance by pulling the outer edges into the centre back.

4 Progress up the back of the head with horizontal sections, each section approximately 3cm deep, combing the hair down to its natural fall. Cut the hair, following the base line as a guide, cleanly and squarely across in a straight line.

5 At the occipital bone take a horseshoe section into the recession area on both sides of the head. Over-direct the side and front sections into the baseline at the back of the hair cut and follow the guide. Work in horizontal sections, up to the profile line; then, when all the sections have been cut, check the balance.

6 From the front at the profile line, take a diagonal back section to the apex of the ear about 3cm deep in the hairline. Work equal distribution on both sides of the head.

7 Combing these sections down to the natural fall, cut a line visually, up from the baseline to nose, lip or chin level. The level at the front depends on the client's preference and also the length of the hair that is being worked with, as a fringe may already be incorporated within the haircut.

8 Cut exactly the same line on the other side of the head and then check the balance by pulling fine sections of hair from key areas on the head into the centre front, cross-checking at the front and working down to the baseline.

9 The next section is taken in a wedge, thicker at the profile line, finer at the apex. This section is combed down to the natural fall and cut using the guide line.

10 Continue working back to the radial section, when both sides have been cut; from the profile line comb all the hair down to the natural fall and check the balance. The outline shape of the haircut is now in place.

11 Starting at the front, take a section approximately 2cm wide on either side of the profile line to the crown. The graduation line at centre front is used as a guide line for the length of the square layers. The profile line is cut squarely across from the centre front back to the crown.

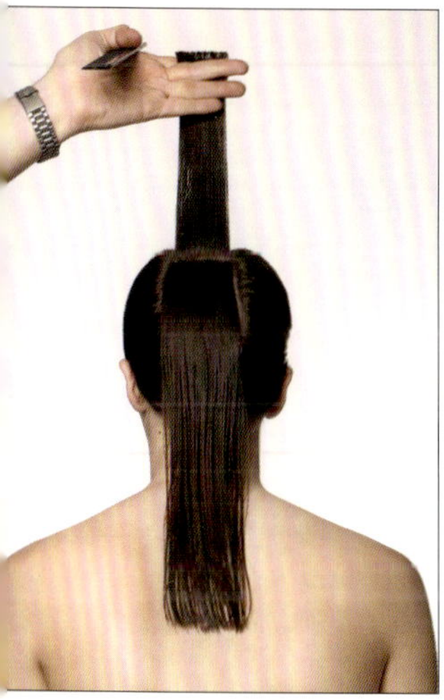
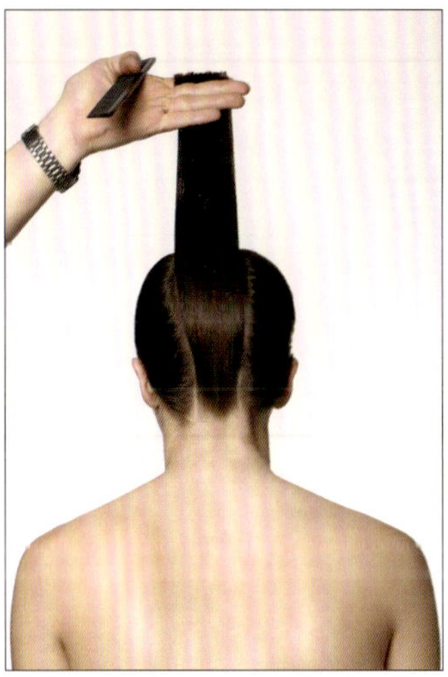
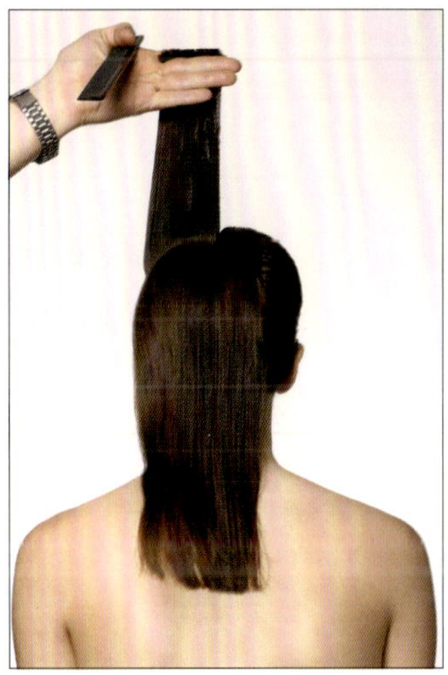
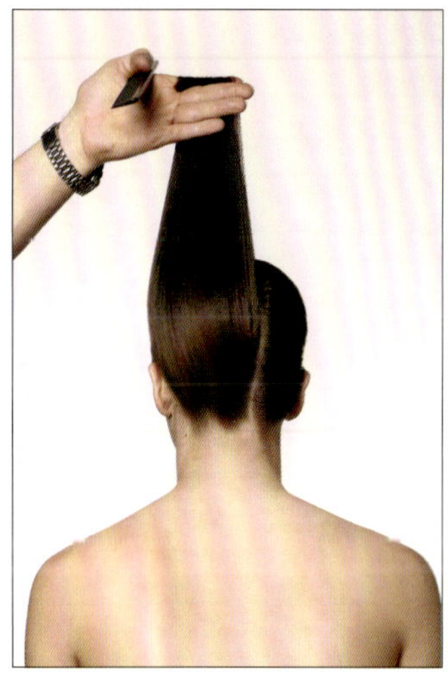

12 Take a horizontal section underneath the profile line at the side of the head, elevate up and over-direct towards the original guide. Continue working down the side of the head and incorporate the front and side hairline, over-directing within the elevation. Repeat the exact same process on the other side of the head. The top and sides of the haircut are now cross-checked by pulling all sections up from the hairline and over-directing up to the profile line.

13 Connect the back to the top by taking a horizontal section 3cm below the crown. Sub-divide this section by making a parting 2cm wide on either side of the profile line. Incorporate the guide line from the crown and square up, cutting across the guide line. Continue working down the centre back of the head by over-directing and squaring up to the guide line. Finish this section at the hairline at the nape. By over-directing up to the crown, length and square layers will be maintained throughout the back of the haircut.

14 Continue with horizontal sections on both sides of the centre back, by squaring up and over-directing to the guide line at the crown. The entire area at the back is cross-checked by pulling sections up from the hairline at the nape and held to the square layer guide line at the crown.

15 The haircut, once cross-checked, is now complete.

16 For the finish, use an appropriate styling product and distribute through the hair evenly. To give body and separation to the hair, the hair can be power dried to use the natural movement and texture of the hair; or if a straight and smooth finish is required, blow dry using a nozzle on the hairdryer and a round metallic brush. Starting at the back of the nape area work around the head in halo sections, direct the hairdryer downward onto the hair and keep a firm tension on the hair for a smooth straight finish.

17 Apply a finishing product to the hair, such as a hair glaze or shine mist. Applied onto the surface of the hair, finishing products promote a smooth finish and healthy shine to the hair.

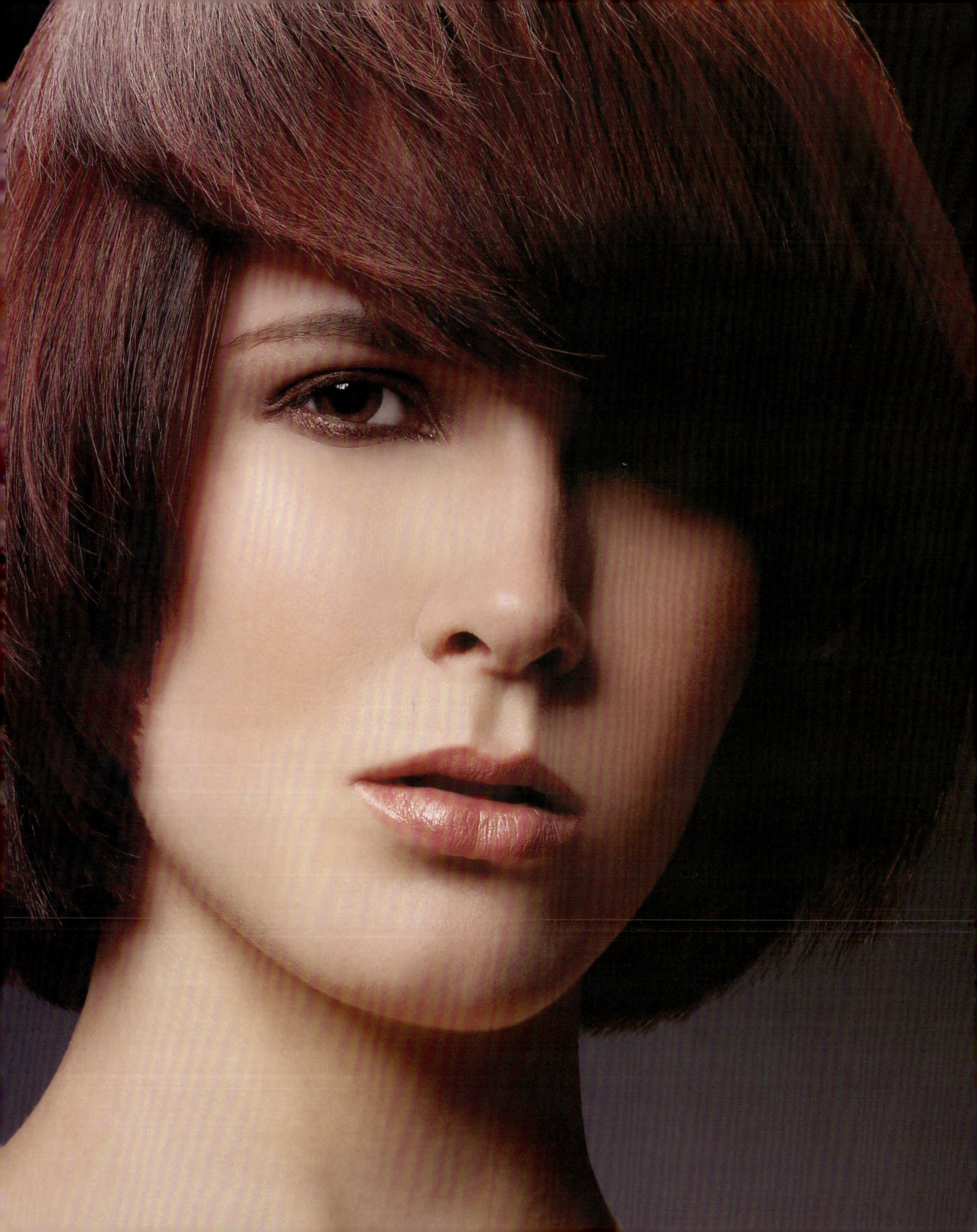

Round Layers

Round layers essentially follows the natural contour of the head – it is a mid-length haircut which eliminates weight in the baseline. The technique employed follows a uniform pattern. Working with the curvature of the head, the shape progresses by pivoting around the crown. Round layers is ideal for most textures, from naturally curly to naturally straight. This haircut is suitable for most face shapes and looks equally good on a man or woman. Surface texture can be achieved by slicing into dry hair, this will break up the shape further and give a seamless finish. At any point on the head, each section should be the same length as the previous one.

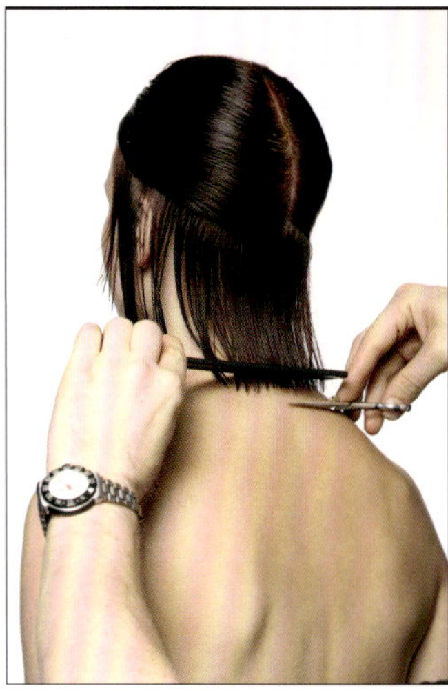
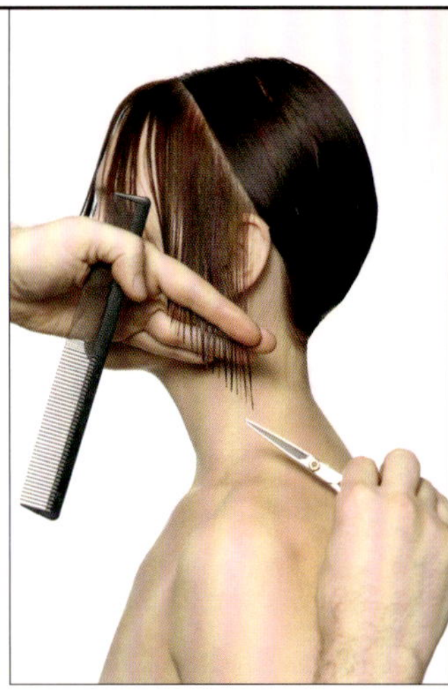
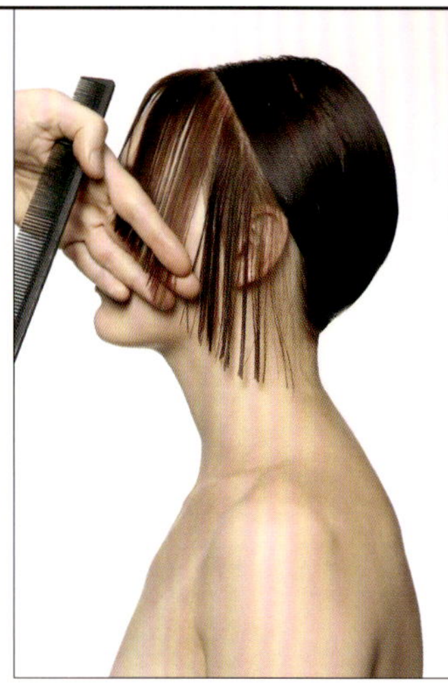
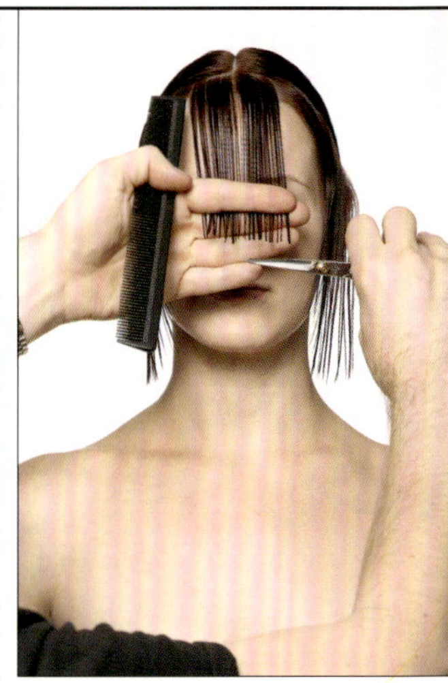

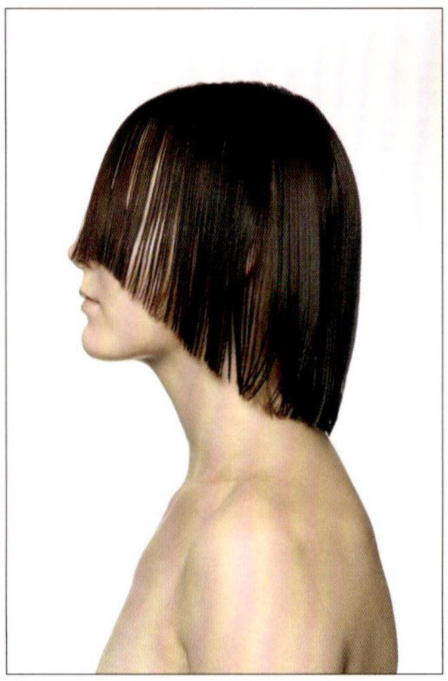
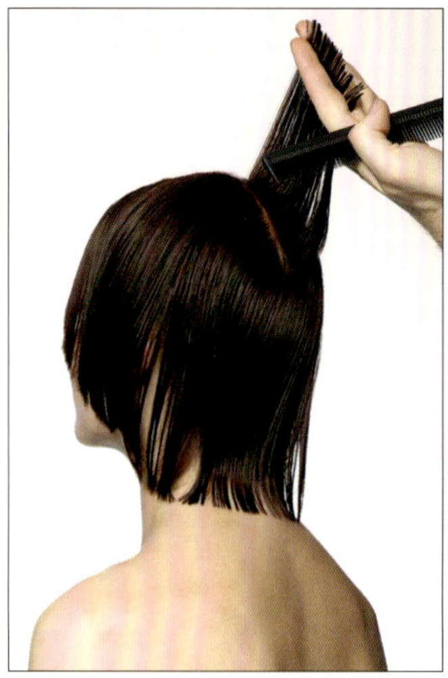
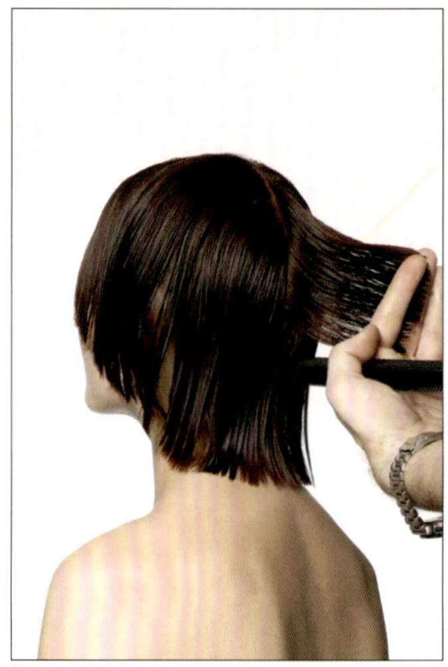
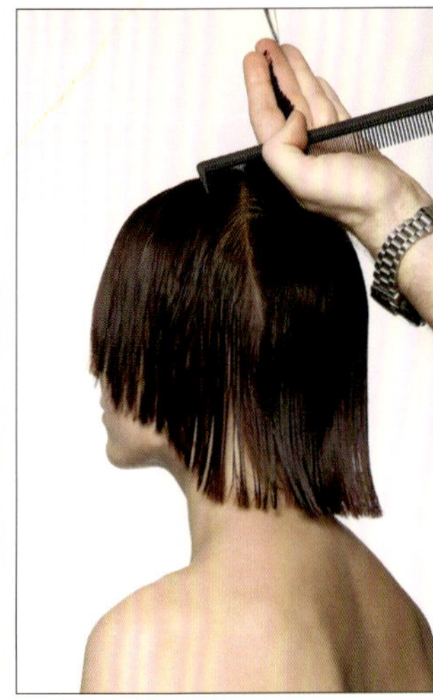

1 For the cut, after shampooing and conditioning, the hair is parted using a halo division which works completely around the head approximately 3cm in from the hairline.

2 Once the length has been determined at the baseline, the baseline length is used as a guide for the length of the layers. The length of the layering remains the same throughout the entire cut regardless of the desired length. This haircut can either be blunt or point cut, depending on the amount of texture required.

3 With the head in an upright position, start the haircut at the centre back of the nape. From the parting at the halo section, comb the hair down to the natural fall using one finger depth elevation and work out to behind each ear.

4 Continue around to the sides and allow for the protrusion of the ear, with one finger depth elevation and the hair combed down to the natural fall. Connect the back into the sides – do this on both sides of the head and check the balance.

5 At the centre front comb the hair down to its natural fall and with one finger depth elevation connect the front into the sides. The guide line and perimeter is now in place.

6 Section off a radial parting. A central vertical section is taken down the centre back of the head from the crown to the nape. Using the pre-determined length at the perimeter as a guide, the layers are cut from the crown to the hairline at the nape and following the natural curvature of the head shape.

7 The layering guide line is now in place. The next section is separated using the crown as a pivot, working in wedge-shaped sections around the back of the head, starting from the centre back and working towards the back of each ear at the radial section. Follow the natural curvature of the head as you progress, holding sections out at a 45 degree angle.

8 Continue the same sectioning pattern on the other side of the head. Cross-check using horizontal sections, working from the crown down the back of the head to the hairline at the nape.

9 From the crown to the forehead, take a section about 1cm wide on either side of the profile line. This section is pulled up at 90 degrees. Connect the back of the haircut from the crown to the front.

10 Using the crown as pivot, the next section is taken in a wedge-shaped section either side of the radial parting. Starting with the crown guide line, the section is pulled out at 90 degrees and follows the curvature of the head, continuing down to the hairline at the side of the head.

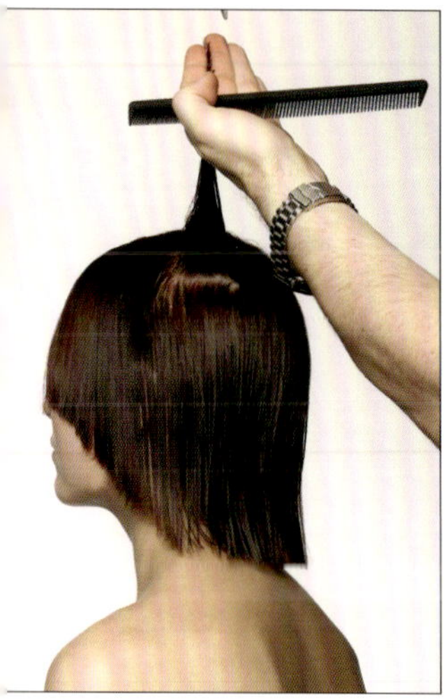

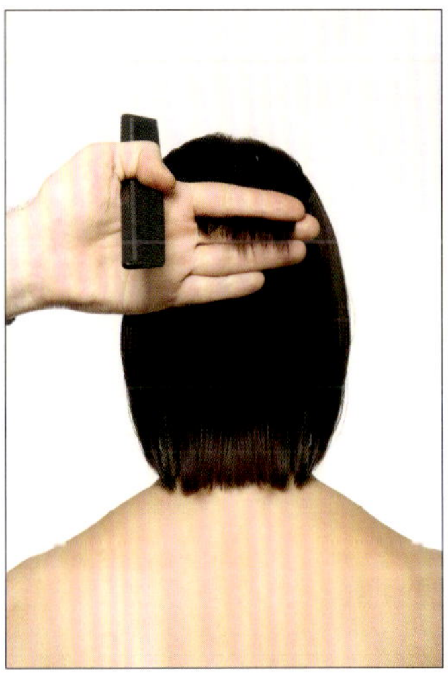

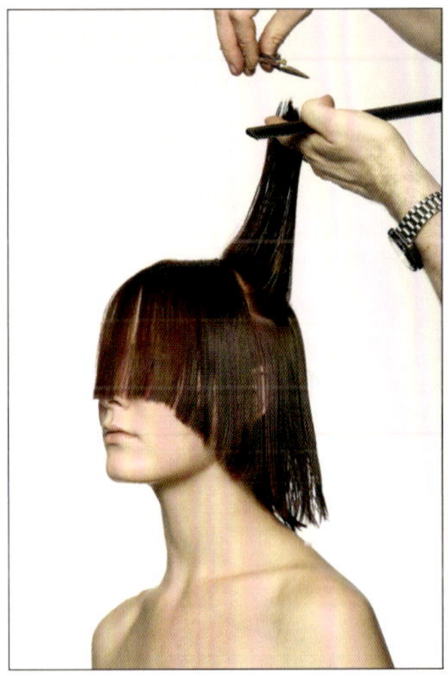

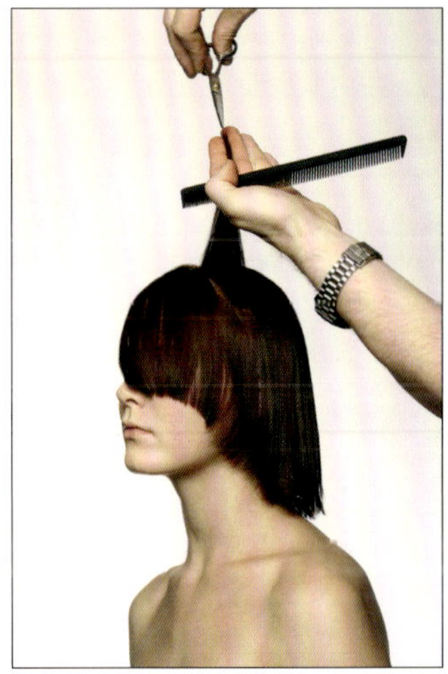

11 Wedge-shaped sections are taken from the profile line to the hairline at the sides and front of the head. Continue to follow the curve of the head.

12 Repeat the same process on the other side of the head. The sectioning pattern used remains the same. Cross-check the balance.

13 The perimeter can now be personalised by point cutting into the baseline, this will soften the edge and eliminate any excess weight.

14 For the finish, use an appropriate styling product and distribute evenly through the hair.

15 Using a hairdryer, the hair can either be power dried for maximum texture and separation; or if a smoother finish is required, blow dry with a nozzle attachment on the hairdryer and use a metallic round brush.

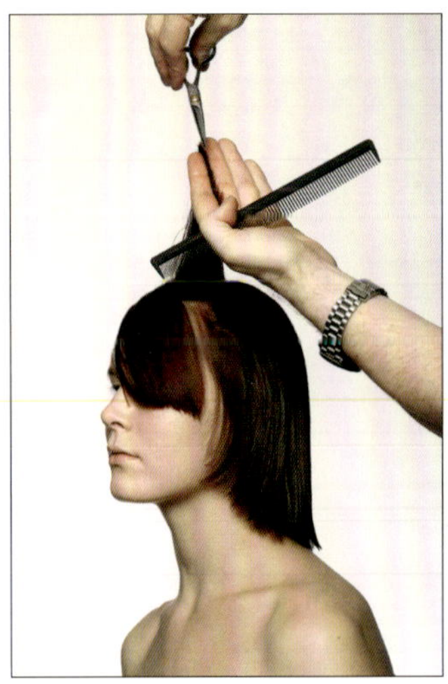

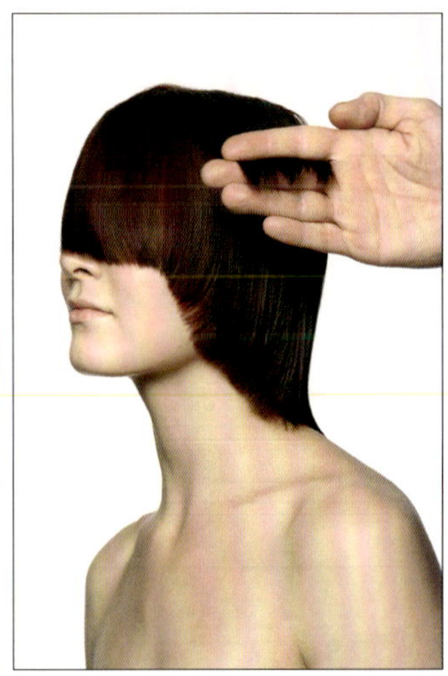

16 Starting at the back of the head, blow dry working around the head in halo, shaped sections.

17 Apply a finishing product to the hair – if the layers are short within the cut work through a hair glaze and apply with the fingers to accentuate texture and separation in the finish.

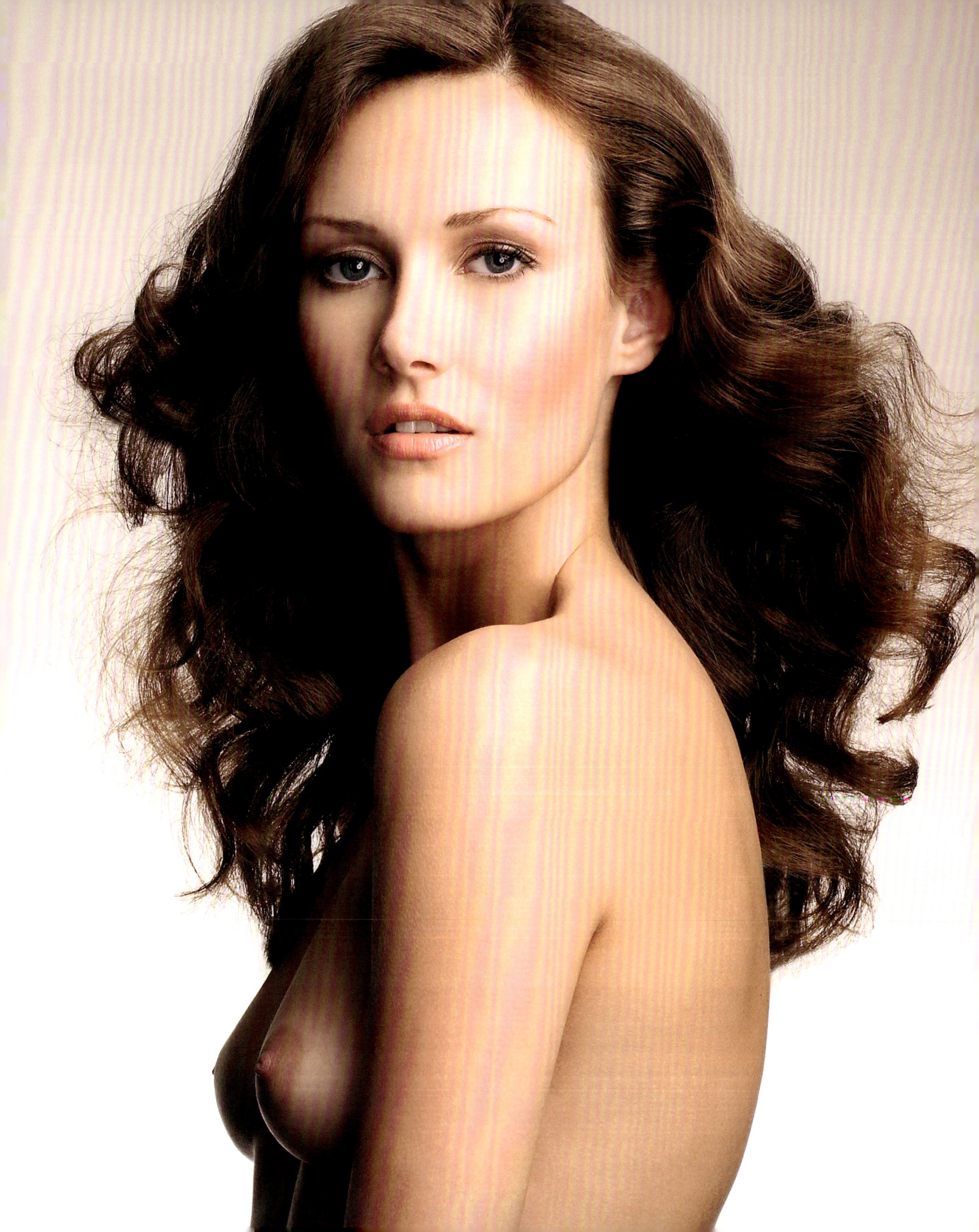

Concaved Layers

The concaved layers haircut introduces a shorter layering pattern around the front of the face while maintaining length throughout the back. This shape works best when it falls below the shoulder. If concaved layers is approached with a pointed into cutting technique this will promote internal volume and texture. Concaved layers revisits the one length with forward graduation techniques and then progresses to an over-directed technique when layering throughout the top sections. This haircut is a pretty and soft feminine shape which is easy to maintain and works well on most textures.

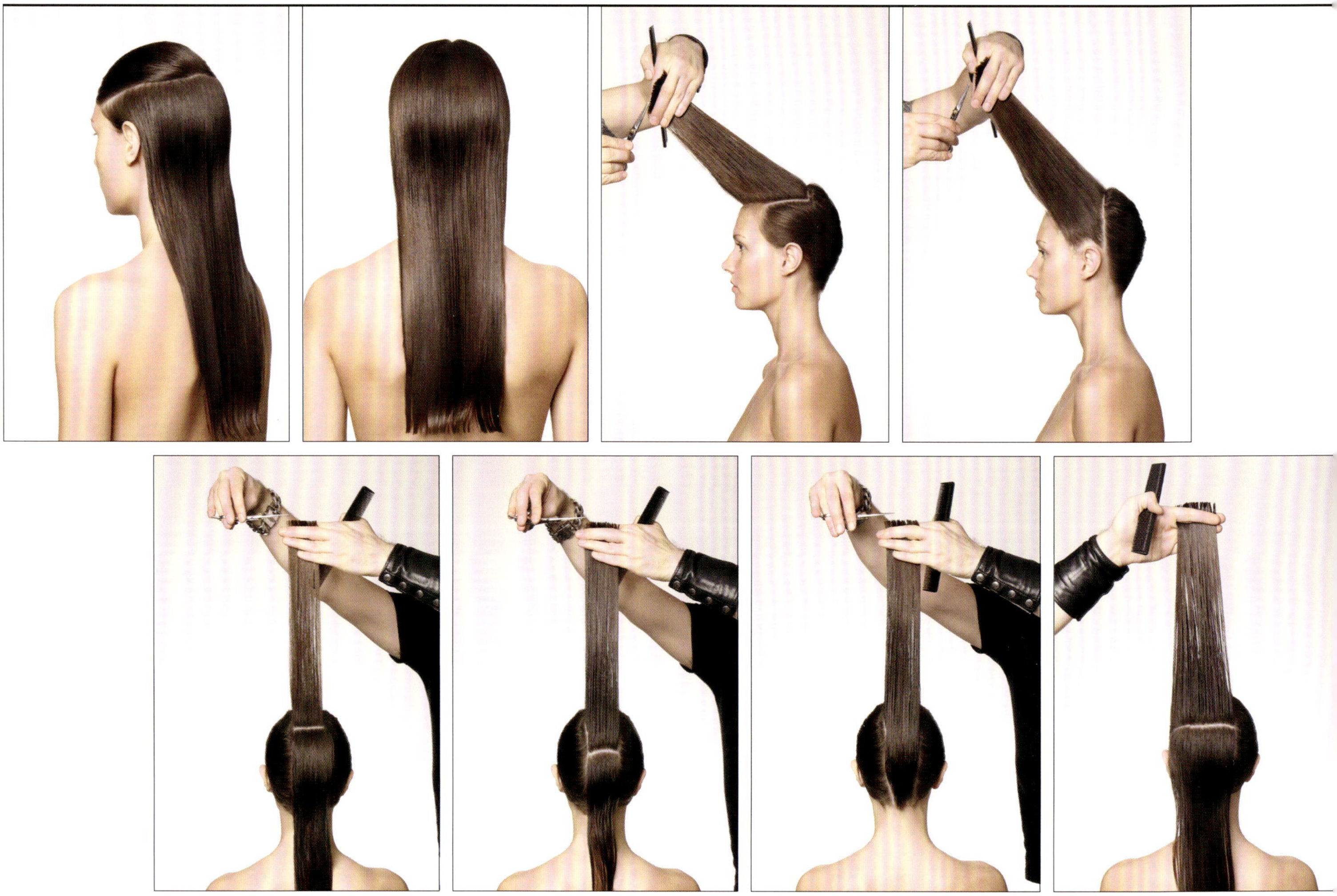

1 For the cut, after shampooing and conditioning, the hair is parted centrally using a profile line from centre forehead to centre nape.

2 With the head in an upright position, two horizontal sections are taken at the nape about 3cm deep, this will depend on the thickness and texture of the hair.

3 The hair is combed down to its natural fall. Working either through the fingers or the comb, the base line is determined. Cut the baseline from the middle at centre back out to each side. Check the balance by pulling the outer edges into the centre back.

4 Progress up the back of the head with horizontal sections, each section approximately 3cm deep, combing the hair down to its natural fall. Cut the hair following the base line as a guide, cutting the hair cleanly and squarely across in a straight line.

5 At the occipital bone take a horseshoe section into the recession area on both sides of the head. Over-direct the side and front sections into the baseline at the back of the haircut and follow the guide. Work in horizontal sections, up to the profile line, then when all the sections have been cut, check the balance.

6 Ideally concaved layers work best shorter at the front and longer towards the back of the haircut, as length and weight is maintained below the shoulder. At the crown take a section approximately 2cm wide on either side of the profile line towards the forehead. Next connect the crown to the front hairline by pulling the hair up at 90 degrees. Starting at the front, the fringe is ignored (if one is in place). On the profile line take a section and cut to about 12cm in length and gradually increase the length, working on a slope back towards the crown. This line becomes the guideline for the proceeding sections.

7 Taking a horizontal section underneath the profile line, elevate up and over-direct up towards the guideline. Continue working down the side of the head and incorporate the front and side hairline, over-directing within the elevation. Repeat the exact same process on the other side of the head. The top and sides of the haircut are now cross-checked by pulling all sections up from the hairline and over-directing up to the profile line.

13 For the finish, use an appropriate styling product and distribute evenly throughout the hair. Power dry to eliminate any excess moisture, then, starting at the nape, blow dry the hair working in the same sectioning pattern as used for the haircut. For a smooth straight finish use a large round metallic brush and direct the hairdryer downward onto the hair and keep a good firm tension on the hair. Personalise the haircut as required.

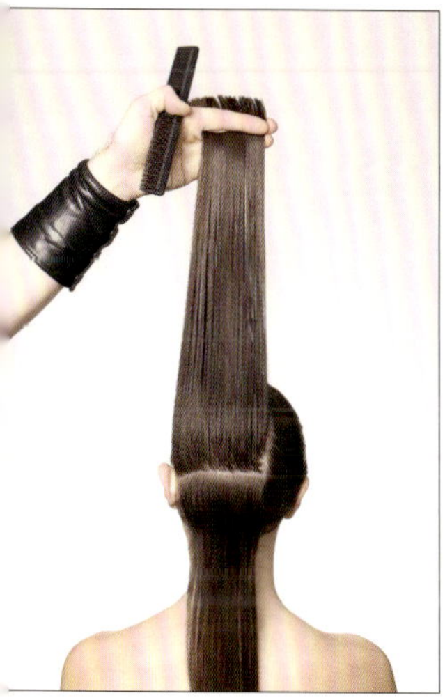
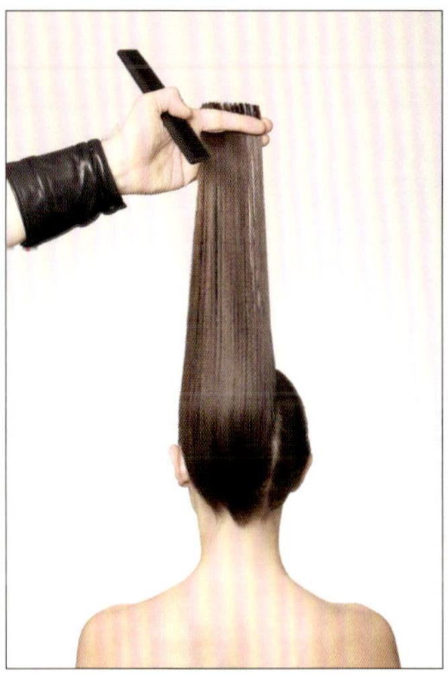
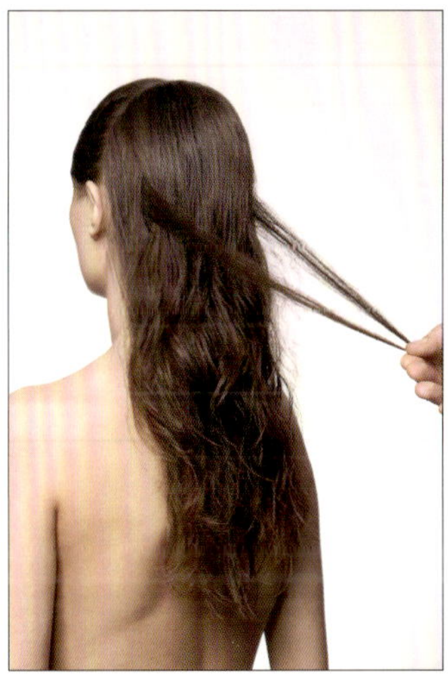
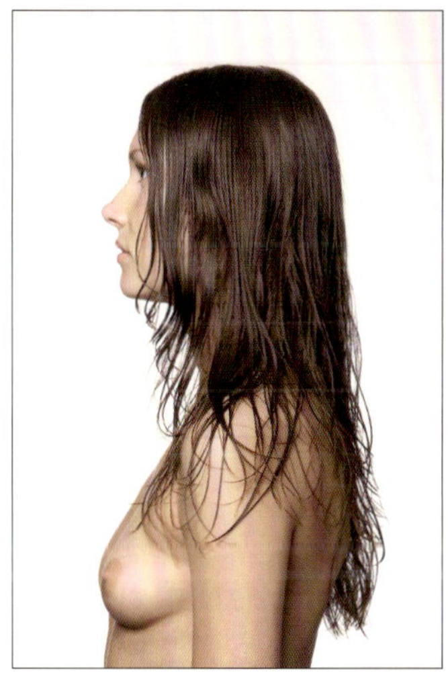

8 From the front hairline at the profile line, take a diagonal back section to the apex of the ear about 3cm deep from the hairline. Work equal distribution on both sides of the head.

9 Comb these sections down to natural fall, and cut a line visually up from the baseline to around lip level.

10 Cut exactly the same line on the other side of the head and then check the balance by pulling fine sections of hair from key areas on the head into the centre front, cross-checking at the front and working down to the baseline.

11 The next section is taken in a wedge, thicker at the profile line, finer at the apex. This section is combed down to the natural fall and cut using the guide line.

12 Continue working back to the radial section, when both sides have been cut. From the profile line comb all the hair down to the natural fall and check the balance. The outline shape of the haircut is now in place and the internal concaved layers are completed.

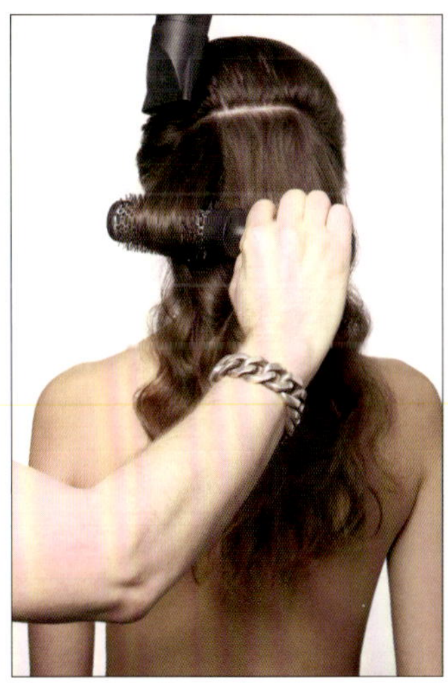
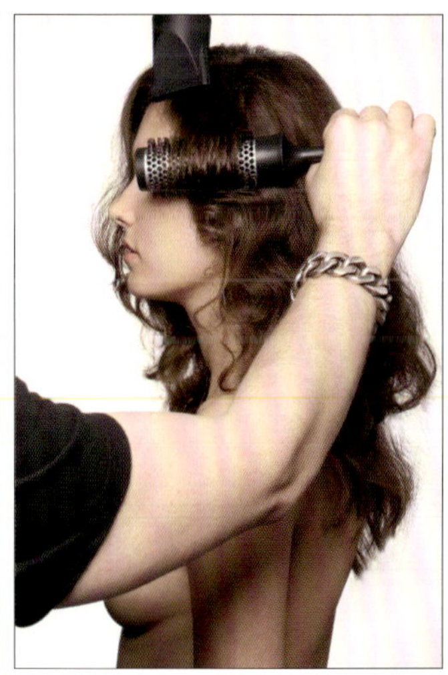

14 Finally, apply a finishing product to the hair, such as a hair mist to give a healthy shine.

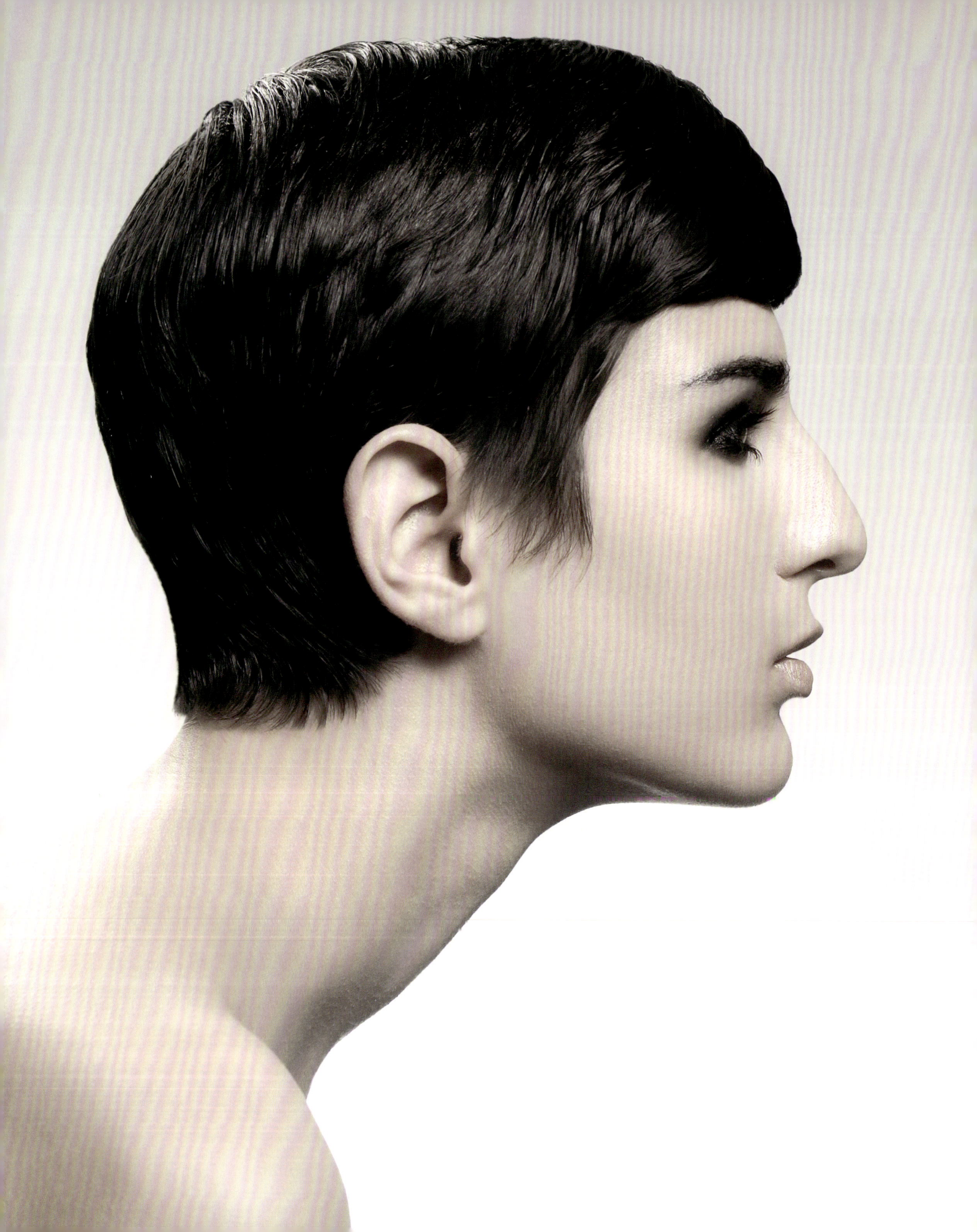

Square Graduation

The square graduation haircut is a truly versatile shape which looks equally as good on a man or woman. To create this shape, begin by working in vertical sections from beneath a horseshoe section by pulling out at a 45 degree angle and progress around the head. Length is maintained through the top sections from the crown towards the front. This short layered shape can be blunt cut for a classic finish or point cut and chipped into to promote texture and separation.

Softness around the ear and nape area gives the woman's version more versatility, while a closer outline gives the man's version a masculine feel.

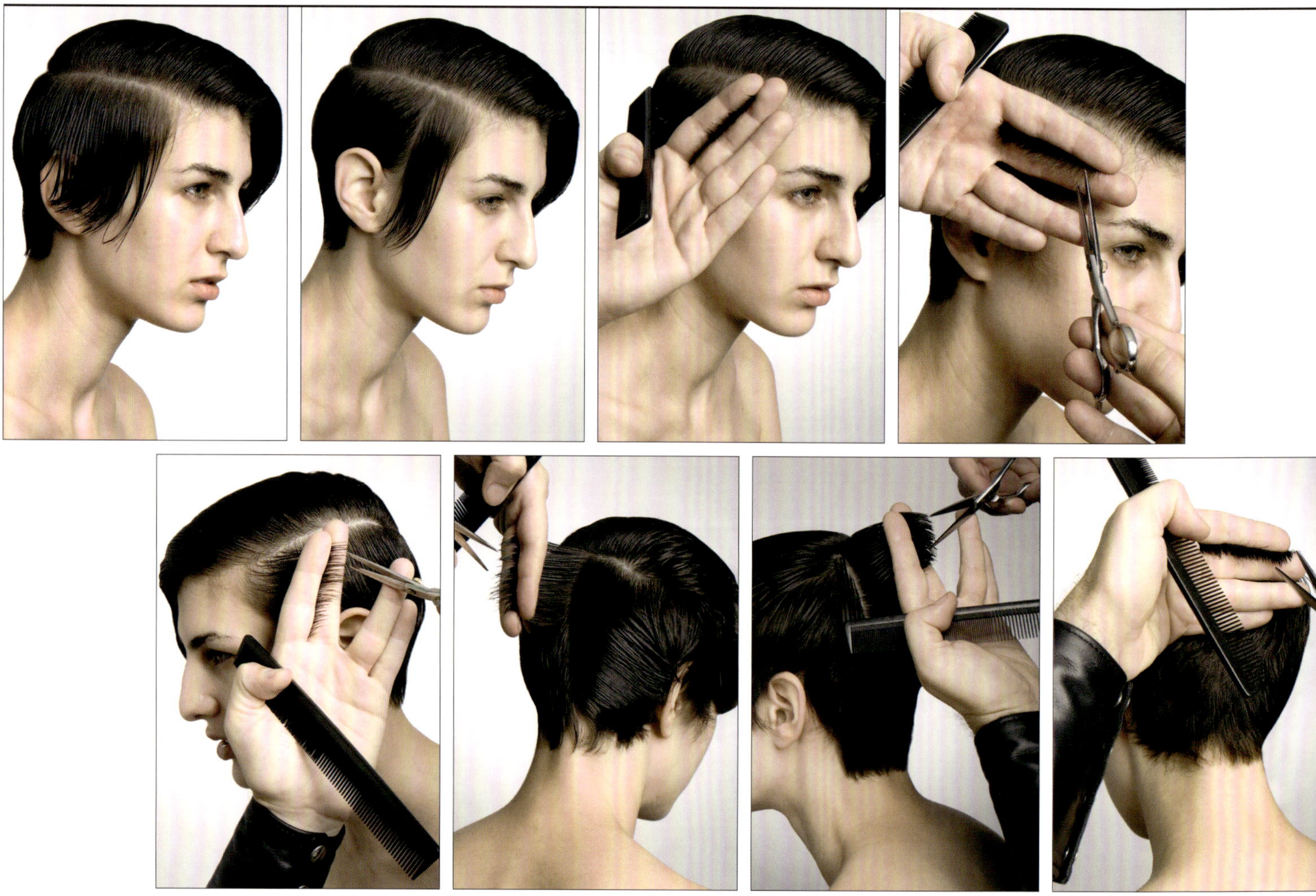

1 For the cut, after shampooing and conditioning, the hair is parted using a horseshoe section which runs from the recession area at the temples, and through the occipital bone at the centre back of the head. Section off the remaining hair on top of the head.

2 With the head in an upright position, on the side of the head at the front hairline, take a vertical section from the horseshoe parting down to the hairline just in front of the ear. Pull out at 45 degrees and determine the length, depending on the required finish; this technique could be blunt or point cut.

3 With the first section in place this now becomes the guideline for each side of the haircut. Continue working in vertical sections using the pre-cut length as a guide on the side of the head. Work as far as the radial section and then cross-check by pulling out horizontal sections.

4 Repeat the exact same process on the other side of the head and then cross-check the balance on both sides of the head.

5 At the centre back take a vertical section from beneath the horseshoe parting down to the hairline at the nape. Pull this section out at 45 degrees and cut the line from the occipital bone to the nape – this section becomes the guide for the back.

6 From the centre back continue working on the right hand side of the head. Take vertical sections around the back of the head out to behind the ear and connect into the side of the haircut. Repeat this procedure on the back left hand side, then cross-check the entire back section by taking horizontal sections ensuring a smooth connection between the sides and the back.

7 The perimeter is then put in place at the back and sides. Comb all the hair down from the horseshoe parting down to the natural fall. Elevate out and point cut if a soft edge is required, or for a stronger outline work through the comb.

8 With the radial section still in place, from the crown take a vertical section down the centre back of the head and pull out at 45 degrees and make a connection from the crown to the occipital bone. On the right hand side of the head continue working around the back of the head and finish at the radial parting then repeat the same process on the left side. Check the entire back section by pulling out horizontal sections to cross-check.

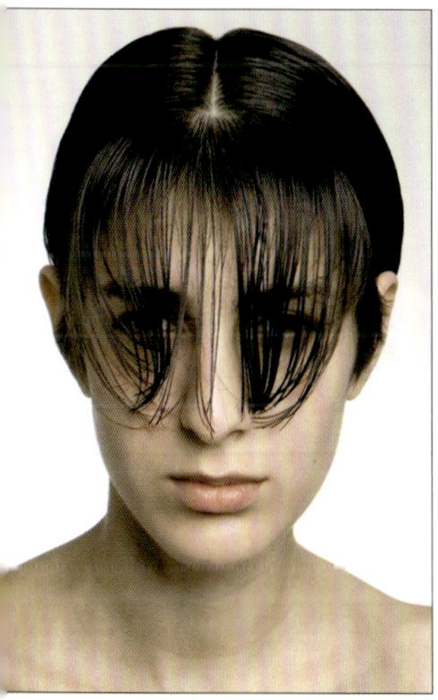
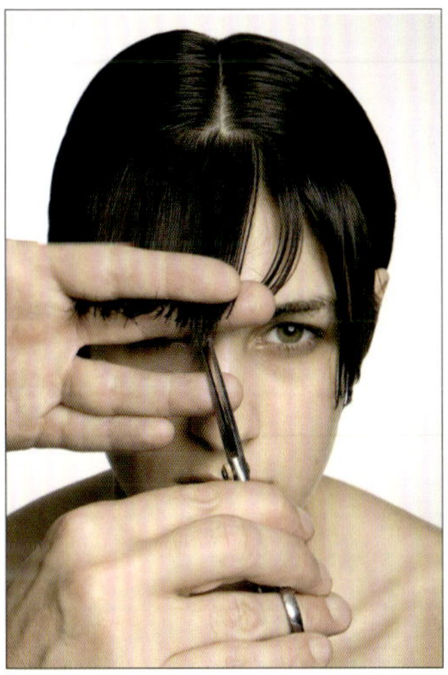
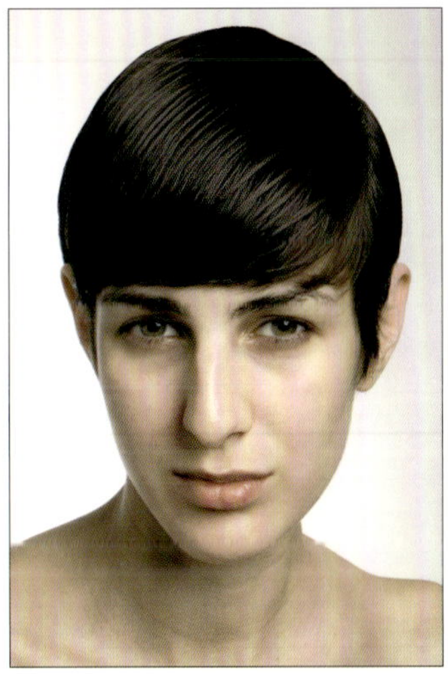
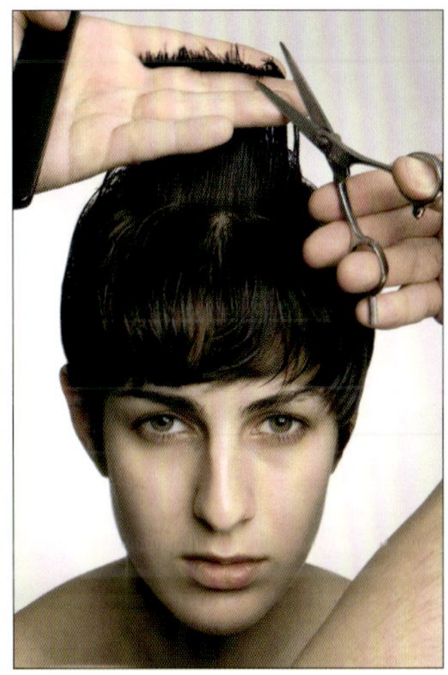

9 At the crown take a section from across the radial parting which incorporates the guide line and pull up to 90 degrees. Cut following the guide.

10 Connect the back of the cut to the top by working from the crown down towards the front hairline, taking sections perpendicular to the sides of the head and pulling up to 90 degrees.

11 The perimeter through the front is then cut and connected into the sides. Cross-check the balance.

12 At the horseshoe section there may appear to be a slight disconnection, this area can be rounded off and any excess weight build-up eliminated.

13 After cross-checking the haircut is complete.

14 For the finish, use appropriate styling product and distribute evenly throughout the hair.

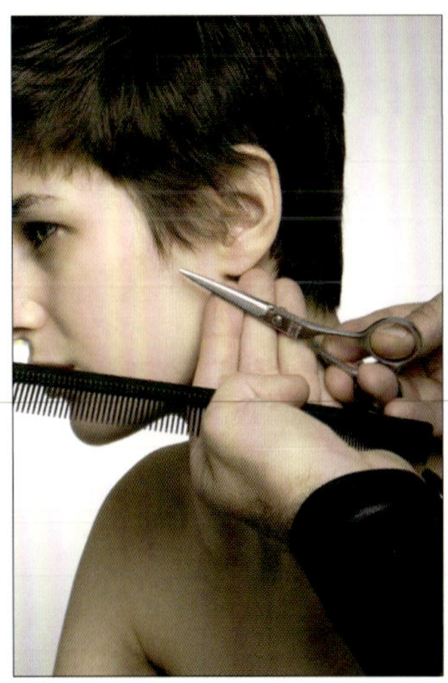
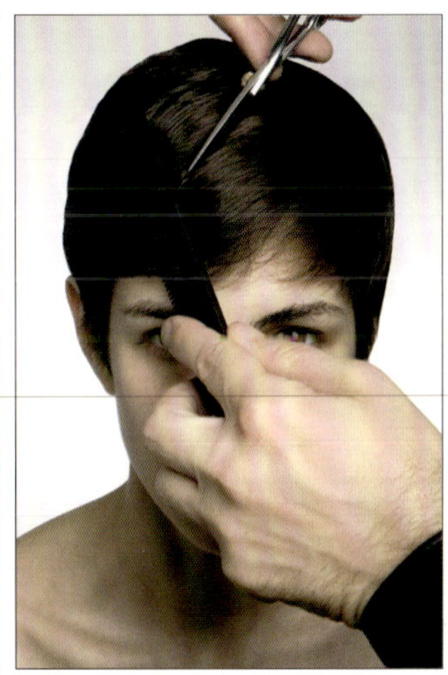

15 Depending on the finish required, the hair can either be power dried by using the fingers or blow dried with your choice of brush.

16 Once the hair is dried, the haircut can be personalised as required. Finally apply a finishing product to the hair to give maximum texture and separation.

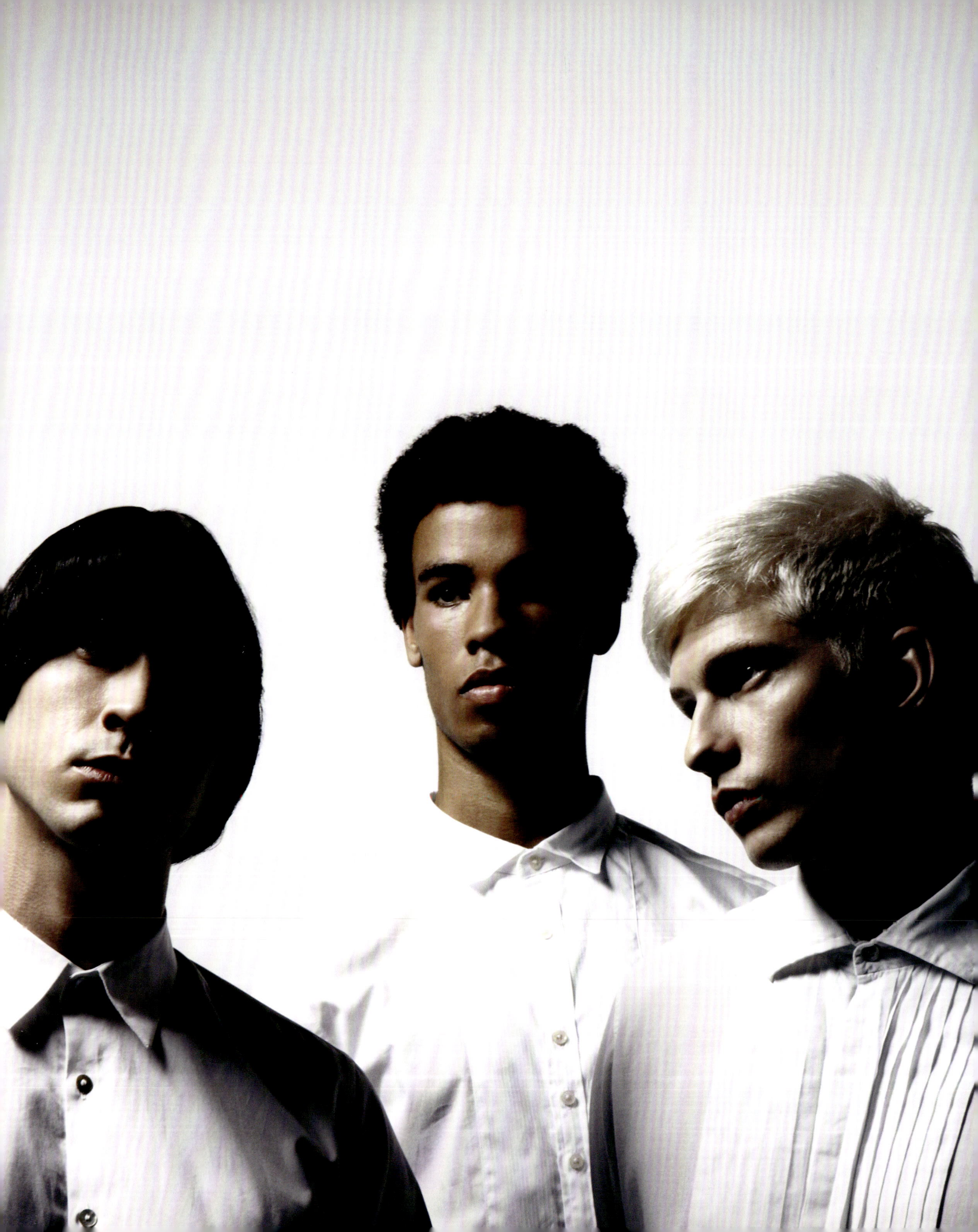

Barbering

Barbering for men focuses on being able to cut various shapes which are usually short, layered and graduated. Barbering and male grooming often incorporates working on beards, moustaches and sideburns.

Technically a man's haircut is usually a graduated shape – accurate graduation creates fine layering. Layering is achieved by taking sections of hair which become an unbroken seamless series of tiny imperceptible lines or layers. The more a section is elevated the greater the amount of layering is made. Layering removes weight as graduation builds weight.

Procedure

Greet and prepare your client.

Discuss your client's requirements.

Examine his hair and scalp and make appropriate recommendations.

Take into consideration hair length, density and texture, shape of face and head.

Determine what needs to be done and make appropriate suggestions.

Decide which cutting techniques will best be used for the desired effect.

With the agreement of your client, then proceed with shampoo and conditioning.

Position client and proceed with the hair cut and finish.

Gowning up correctly is very important before any service. Give a thorough consultation and confirm the service with your client. Work on newly shampooed hair so that the hair and scalp are clean and all styling products have been removed. Use a cutting collar. Position yourself so you are at the correct height for the client, keeping your back straight. Position your client, making sure that he is sitting upright without his legs crossed, and that his head is in an upright position.

Neck brushes may be used throughout the service to remove hair from the face and neck. Always change a disposable razor blade in front of the client so that your hygiene practices can be observed. Take care to ensure the hair line around the ears is clean if the ears are exposed – use clippers on the neck to remove hair. Once the haircut is complete take the client to the backwash and rinse his hair, this will eliminate any hair clippings. Style, finish and clean up using a neck brush. Always ask the client if he is happy with the result.

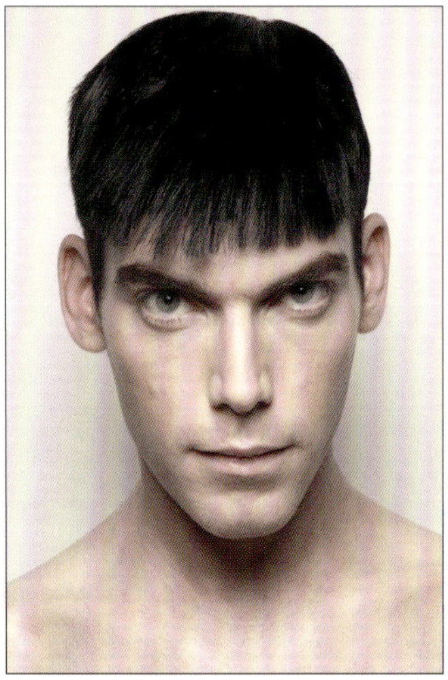
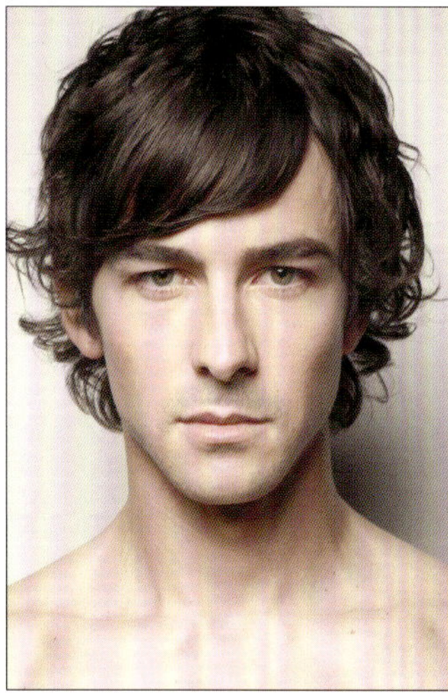
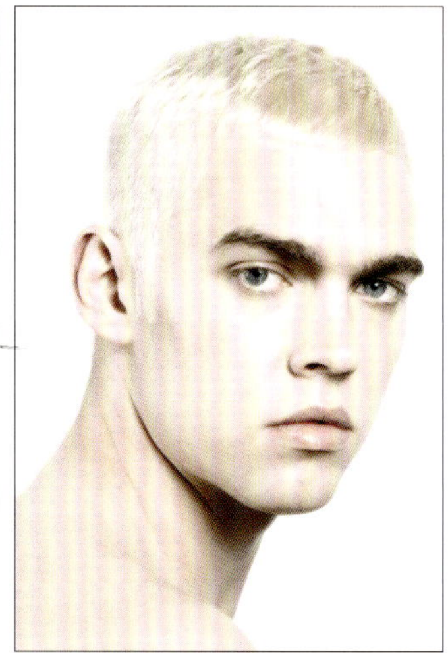
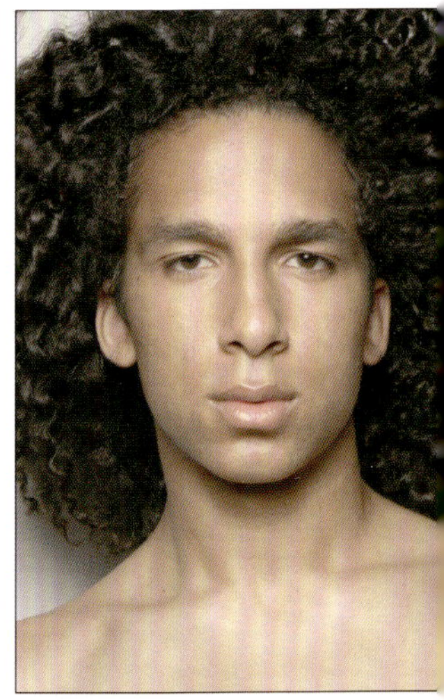
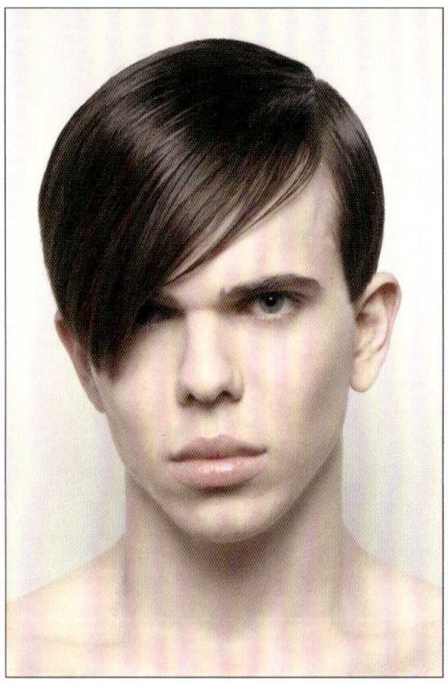
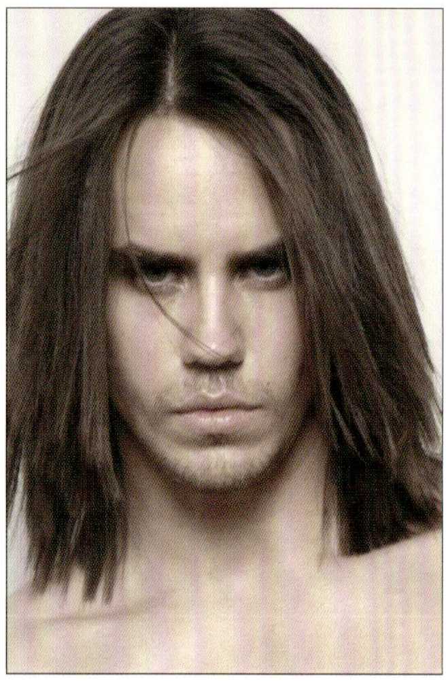
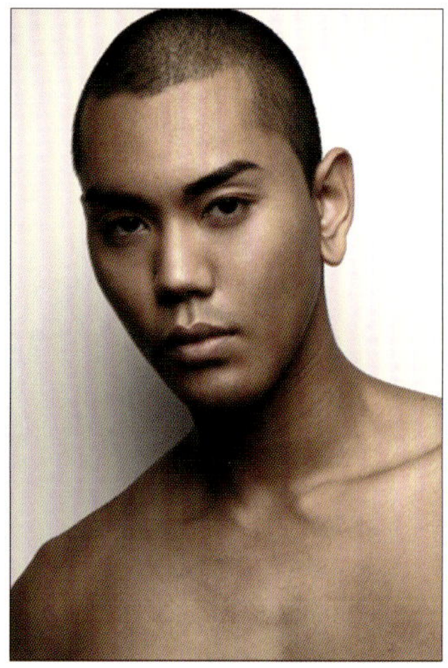
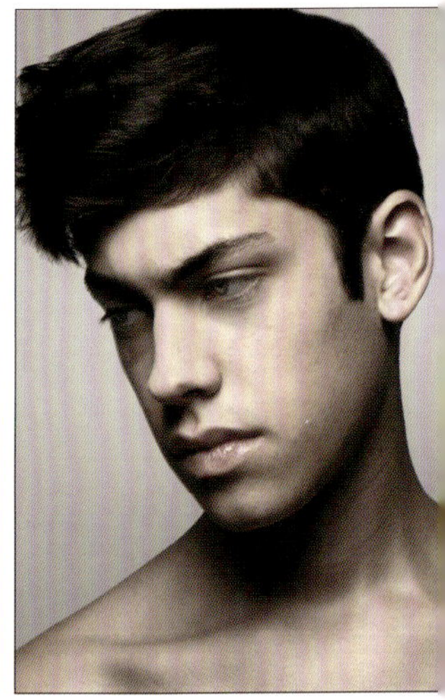
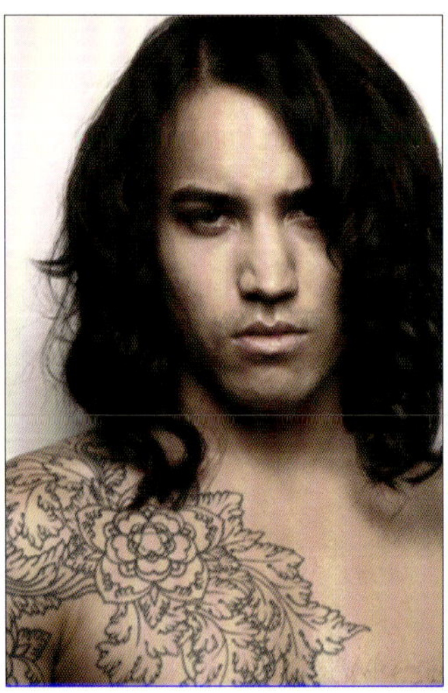
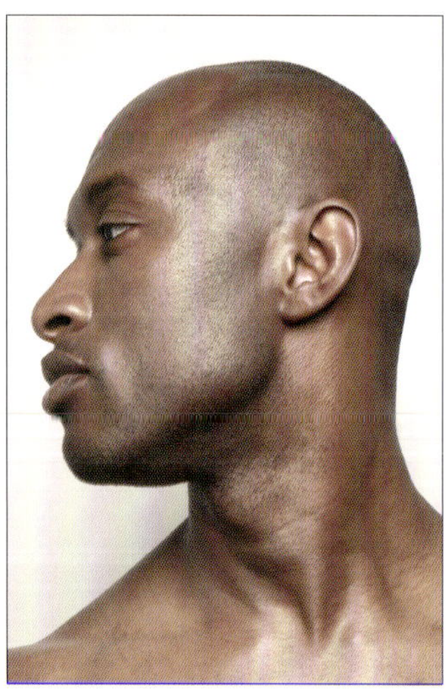
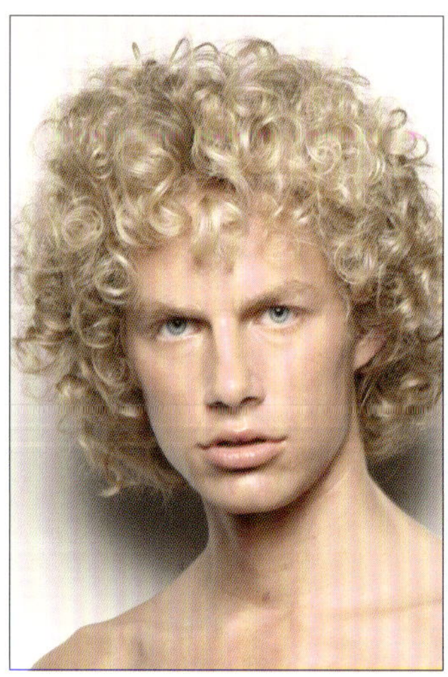
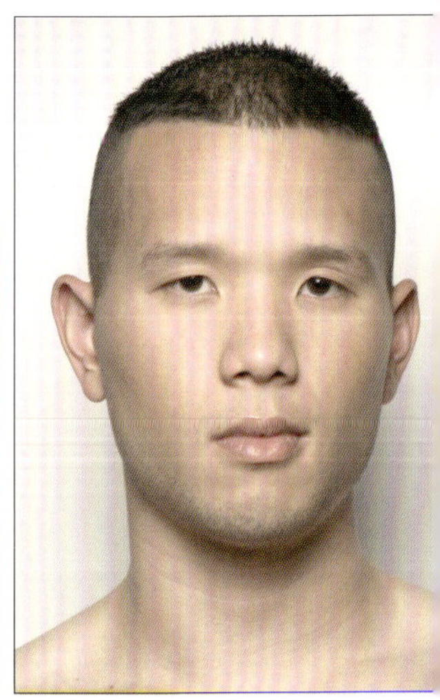

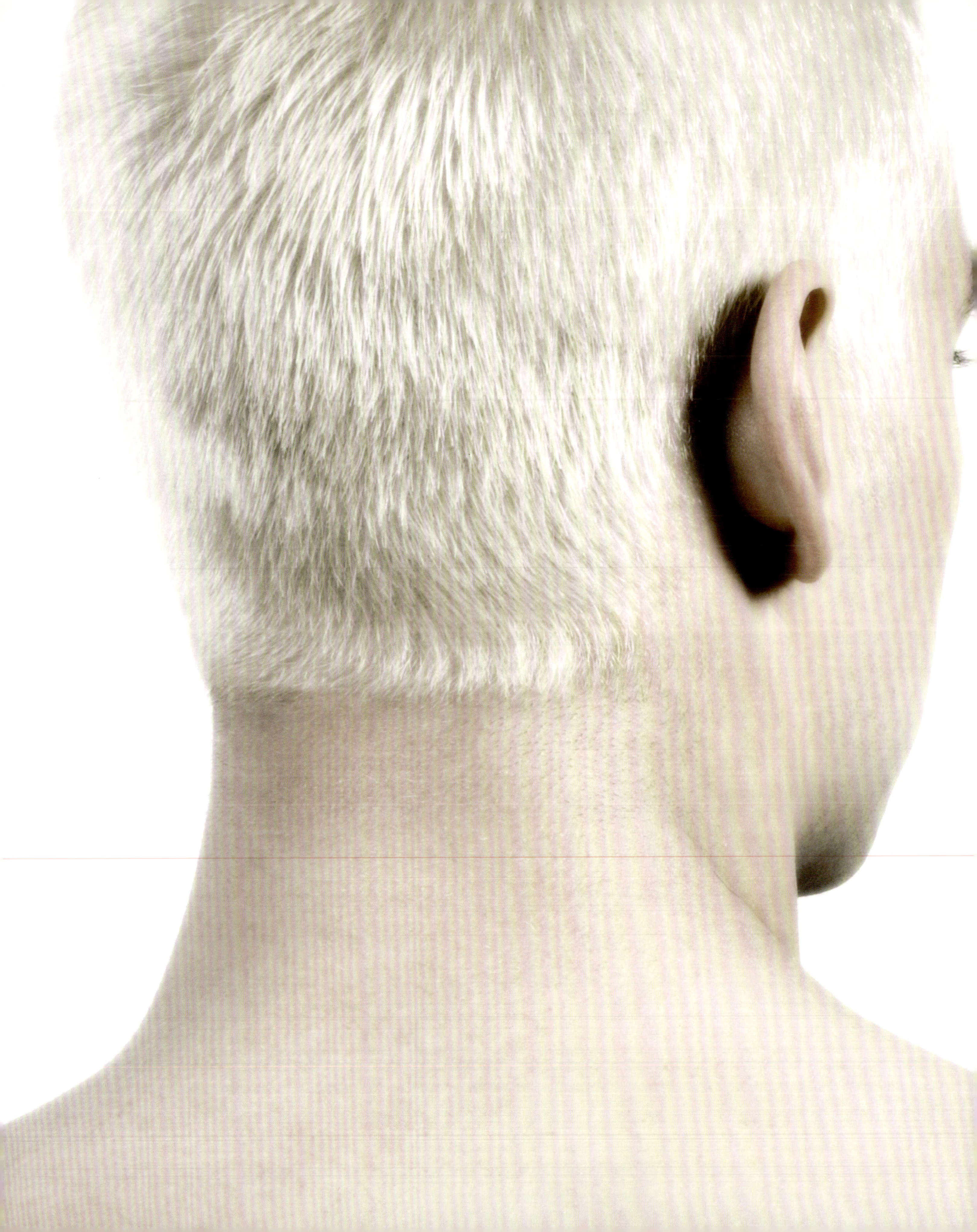

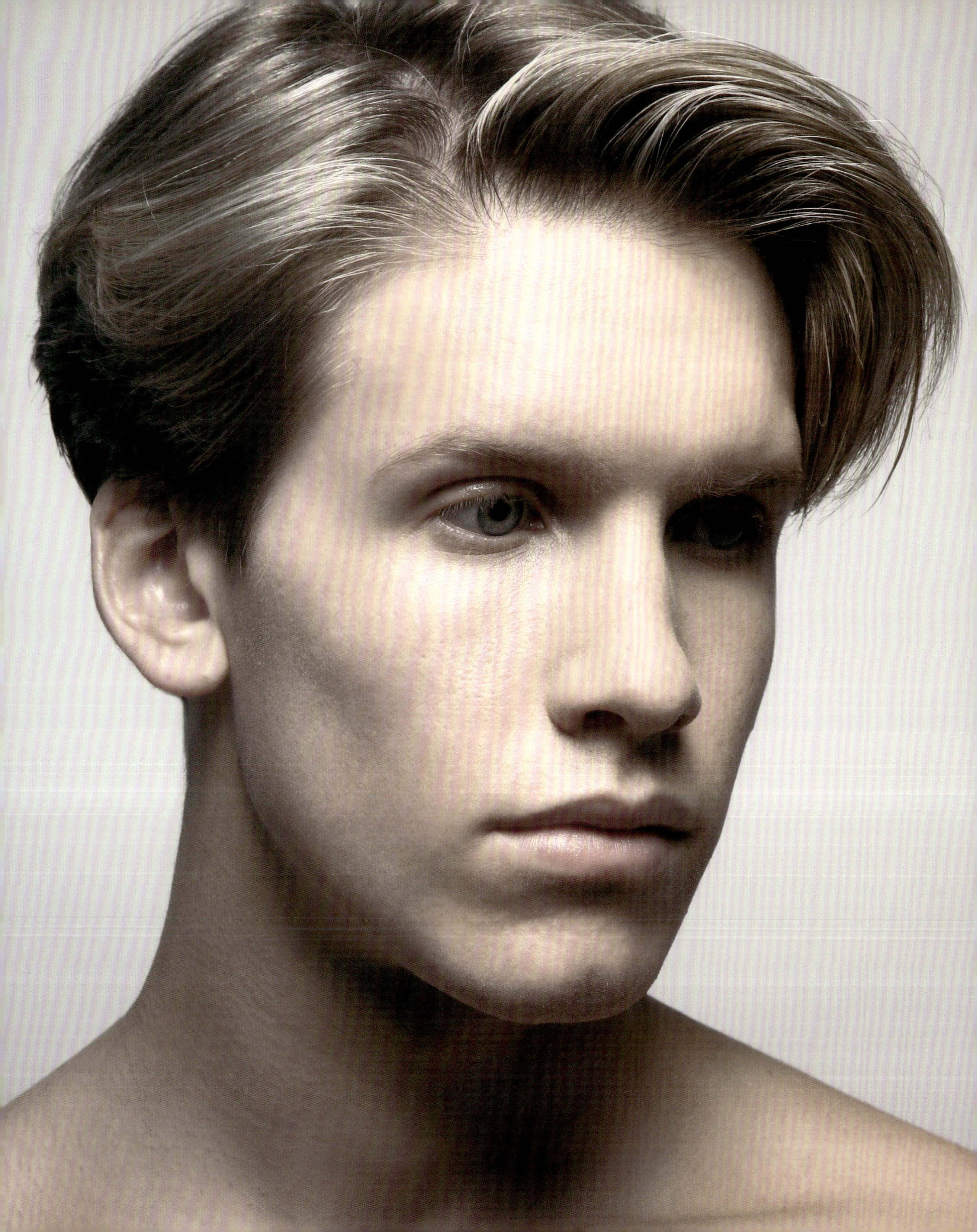

Stretch Graduation

Stretch graduation derives from the haircut commonly known as short back and sides. Graduation is tightly worked through the sides and into the nape area, gradually increasing in length. A very clean shape, which maintains length throughout the top sections, usually incorporates a heavy fringe which can be worked away from the face or left to flop over the eye. It is a versatile masculine shape which remains eternally stylish.

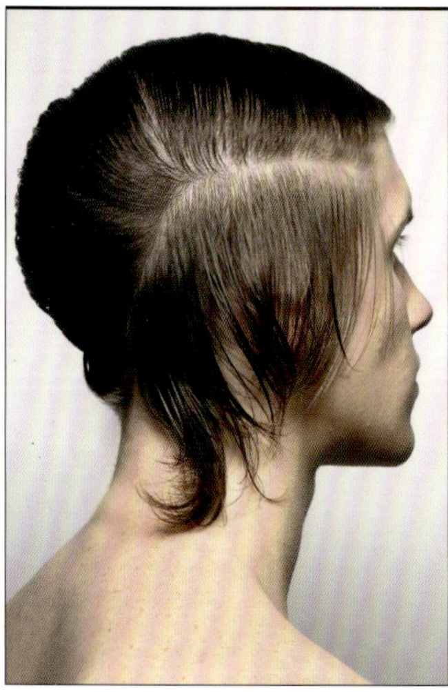
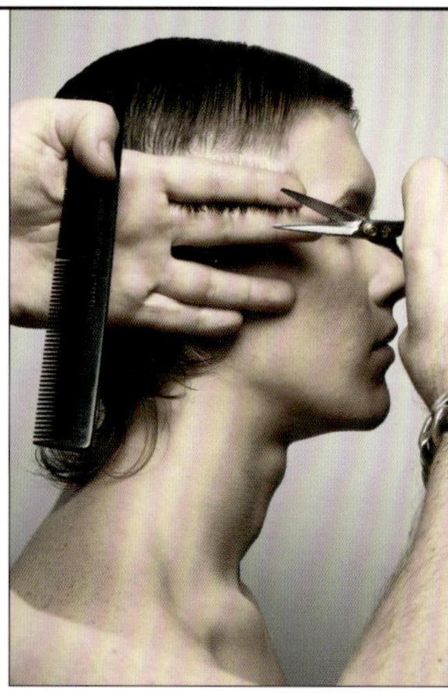
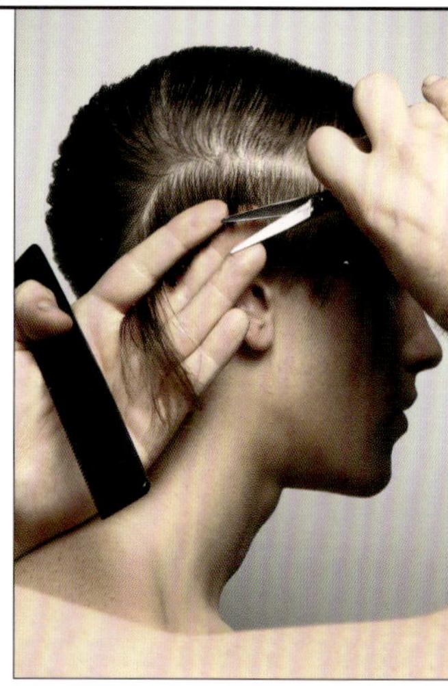

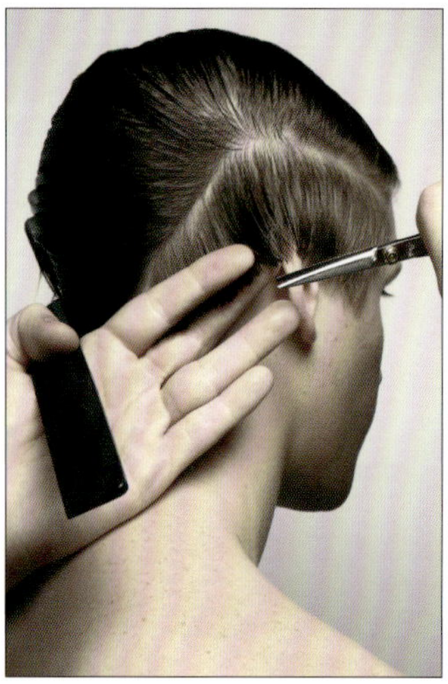
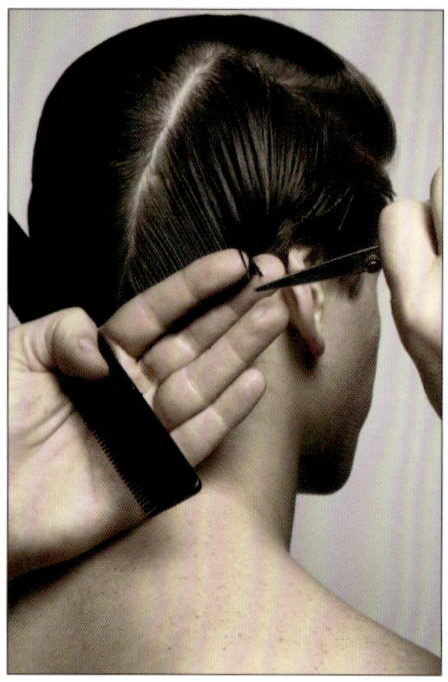
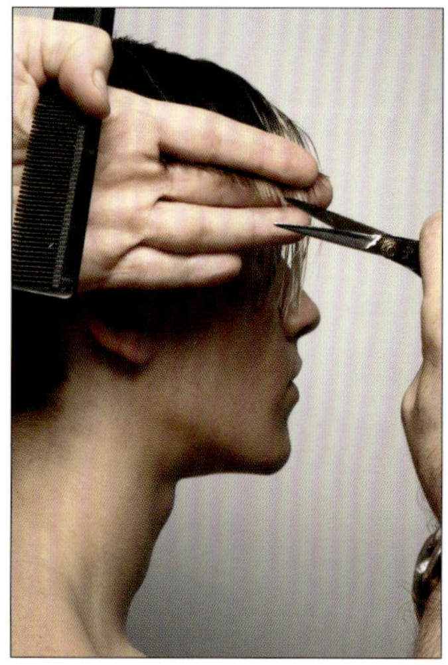
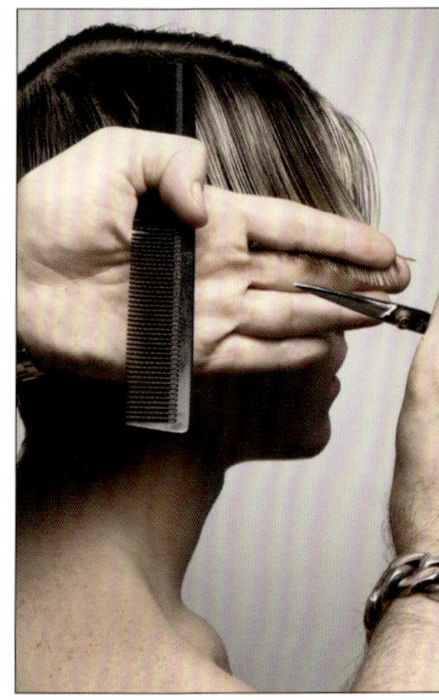

1 For the cut, after shampooing and conditioning the hair, a curved back section is taken from the front hairline and through to the nape area at the back of the ear, usually around 3cm deep depending on the thickness of the hair.

2 With the head in an upright position, elevate out the section at 45 degrees with one finger depth elevation; and determine the length using a point or blunt cutting technique, depending on the amount of texture required.

3 Working away from the face, follow the curve of the head along the side of the head and above the ear, through the section towards the hairline in the nape. Again determine the required length, keeping the proportions the same.

4 The guide line is now in place. Take another section just above the previous one and elevate out at 45 degrees following the curved back section from the front to the nape.

5 Work up the head from the side and side back, curving the line from the front hairline to the nape. All of this section is pulled out to the same level as the guide line to achieve the same level of graduation as the underneath section. The line is continued across.

6 Sections are continued up the head and each section is pulled out and cut, graduation is achieved by following the guideline.

7 Progress up the head to a central profile line which extends from the centre forehead to centre back at the nape.

8 Then starting on the other side of the head repeat the process in the exact same way.

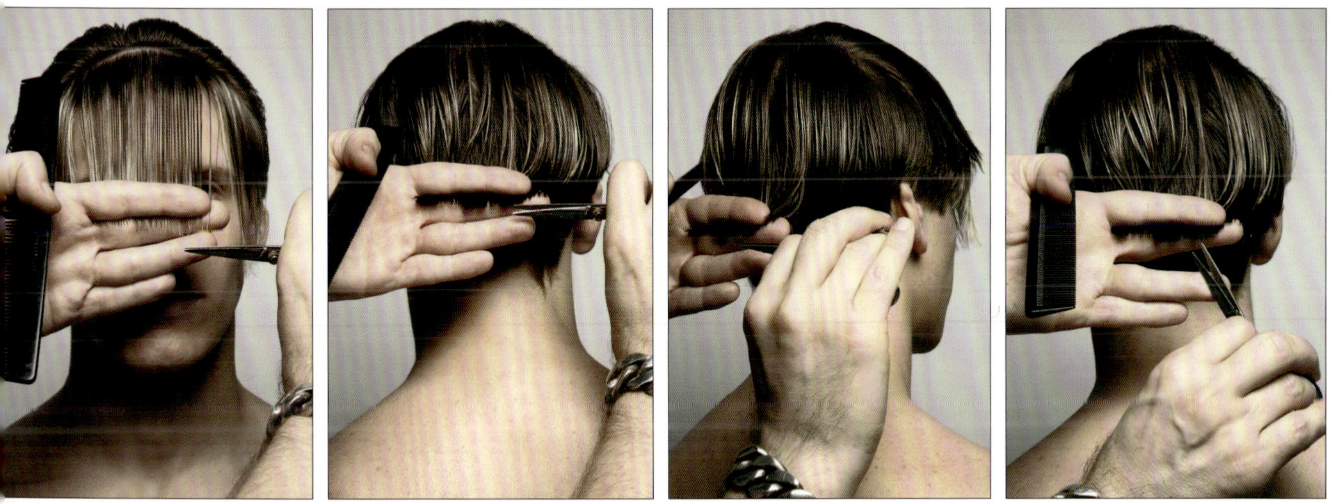

9 On the front hairline take a section around 3cm deep from each recession area, comb down to natural fall and determine the line, remember to keep in proportion with the shape. Take the next section until there is no more hair to cut.

10 At the nape area at the centre back of the head on the hairline, elevate out at 45 degrees and cut across horizontally. This will connect the two sides together and remove a corner previously created by the graduation, progress up to the occipital bone to build weight around that area if desired.

11 Depending on the length required, the hairline through the sides and back can be cut using scissor- or clipper-over-comb techniques and a blend achieved.

12 The stretch graduation cut is now complete. If weight from the top section needs to be removed, simply work horizontal sections across the top of the head and elevate up to 90 degrees from the crown to the front hairline and reduce the weight and length, usually by pointing into the hair to achieve a natural blend. Cross-check the balance.

13 To blow dry, use an appropriate styling product and distribute through the hair evenly. Finger dry for a natural look, or use a vent brush for a more groomed look. Finish with a light pomade, wax or gel.

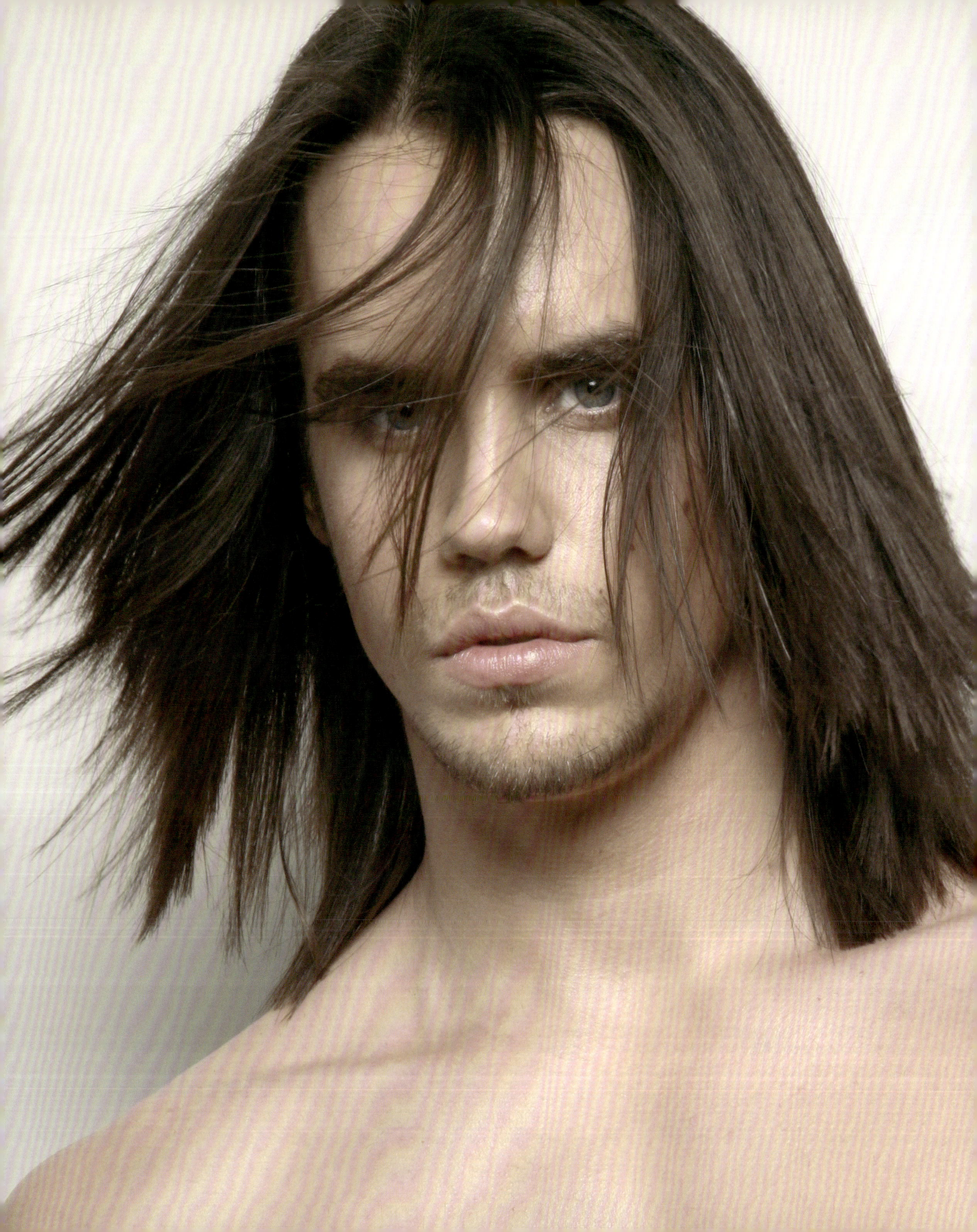

Round Layers

Round layers essentially follows the natural contour of the head – it is a mid-length haircut which eliminates weight in the baseline. The technique employed follows a uniform pattern. Working with the curvature of the head, the shape progresses by pivoting around the crown. Round layers is ideal for most textures, from naturally curly to naturally straight. This haircut is suitable for most face shapes and looks equally good on a man or woman. Surface texture can be achieved by slicing into dry hair, this will break up the shape further and give a seamless finish. At any point on the head, each section should be the same length as the previous one.

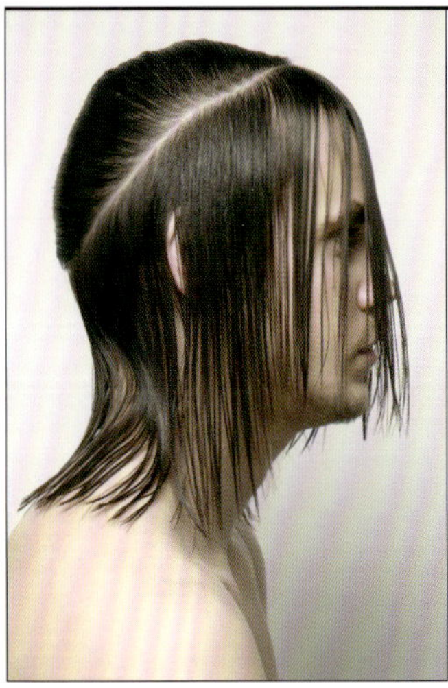
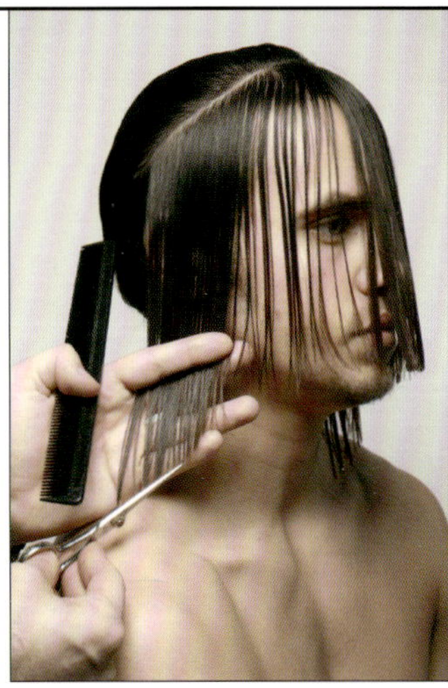
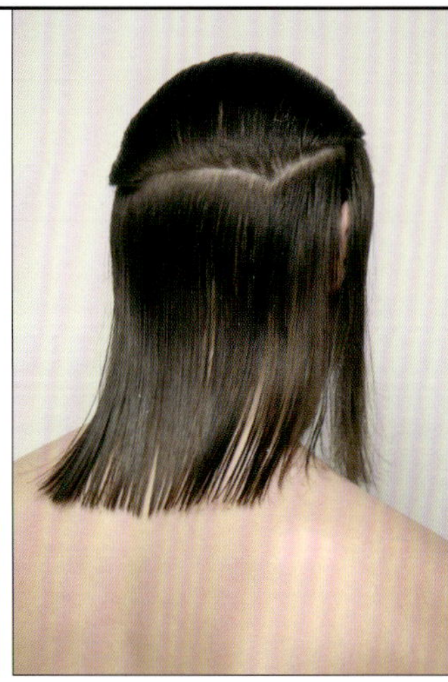
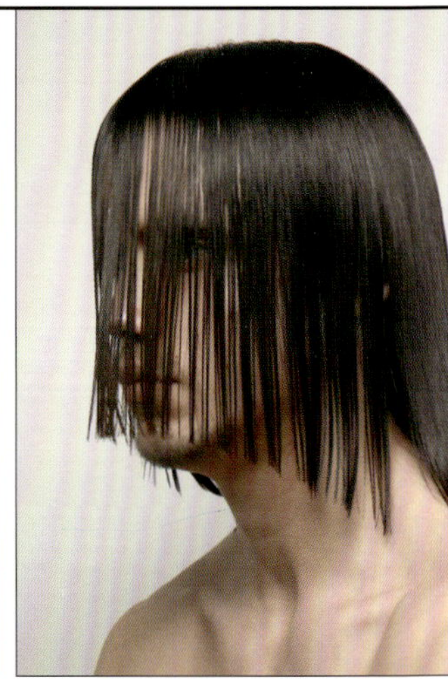
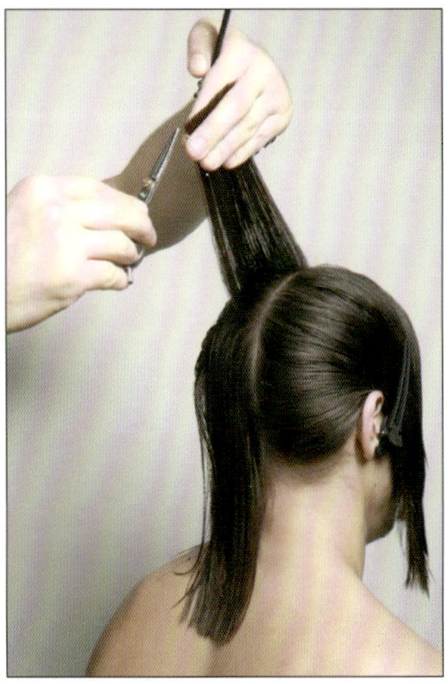
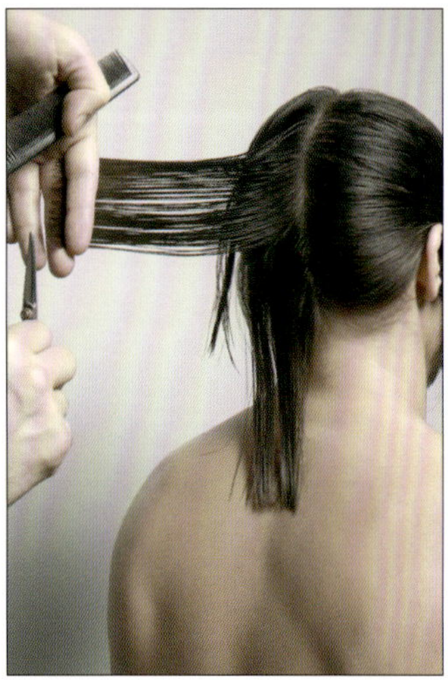
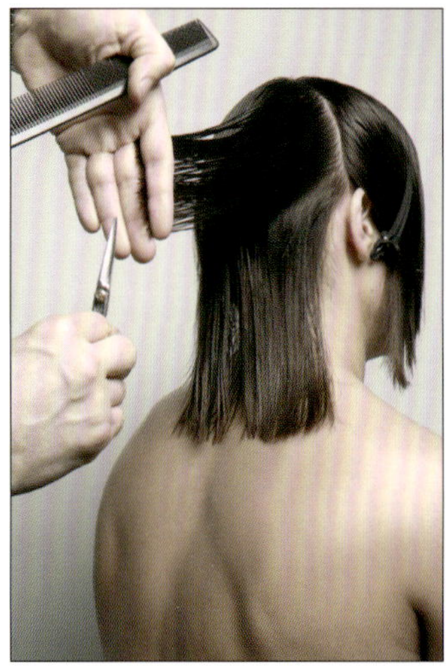
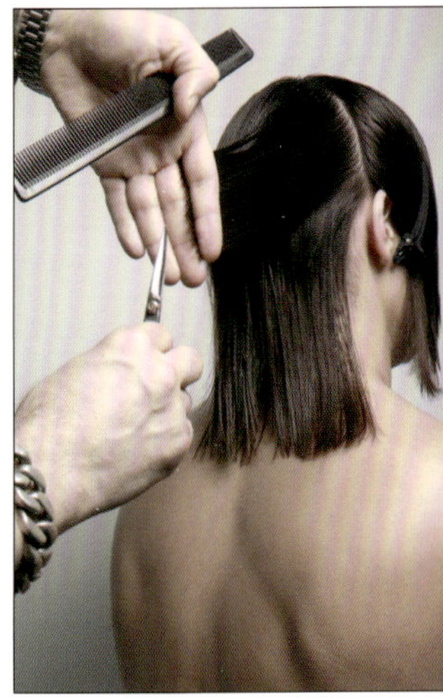

1 For the cut, after shampooing and conditioning, the hair is parted using a halo division which works completely around the head approximately 3cm deep from the hairline.

2 Once the length has been determined at the baseline, the baseline length is used as a guide for the length of the layers. The length of the layering remains the same throughout the entire cut regardless of the desired length. This haircut can either be blunt or point cut, depending on the amount of texture required.

3 With the head in an upright position, start the haircut at the centre back at the nape. From the parting at the halo section comb the hair down to the natural fall and cut using one finger depth elevation, and work out to behind each ear.

4 Continue around to the sides and allow for the protrusion of the ear, with one finger's depth elevation, the hair is combed down to the natural fall. Connect the back into the sides – do this on both sides of the head and check the balance.

5 At the centre front, comb the hair down to its natural fall and, with one finger depth elevation, connect the front into the sides. The guide line and perimeter is in place.

6 Section off a radial parting. A central vertical section is taken down the centre back of the head from the crown to the nape. Using the pre-determined length at the perimeter as a guide, the layers are cut from the crown to the hairline at the nape and following the natural curvature of the head shape.

7 The layering guide line is now in place, the next section is separated using the crown as a pivot, working in wedge shaped sections around the back of the head. Start from the centre back and work towards the back of each ear at the radial section. Follow the natural curvature of the head as you progress, holding sections out at a 45 degree angle.

8 Continue the same sectioning pattern on the other side of the head. Cross-check using horizontal sections, working from the crown down the back of the head to the hairline at the nape.

9 From the crown to the forehead, take a section about 1cm wide either side of the profile line. This section is pulled up at 90 degrees. Connect the back of the haircut from the crown to the front.

10 Using the crown as pivot, the next section is taken in a wedge-shaped section either side of the radial parting. Starting with the crown guide line, the section is pulled out at 90 degrees and follows the curvature of the head. Continue down to the hairline at the side of the head.

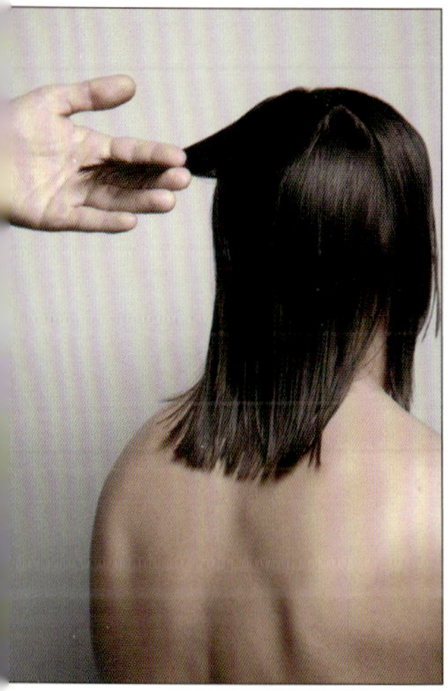

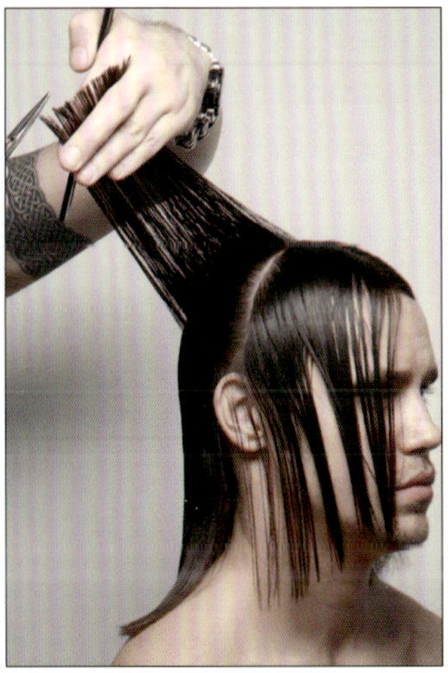

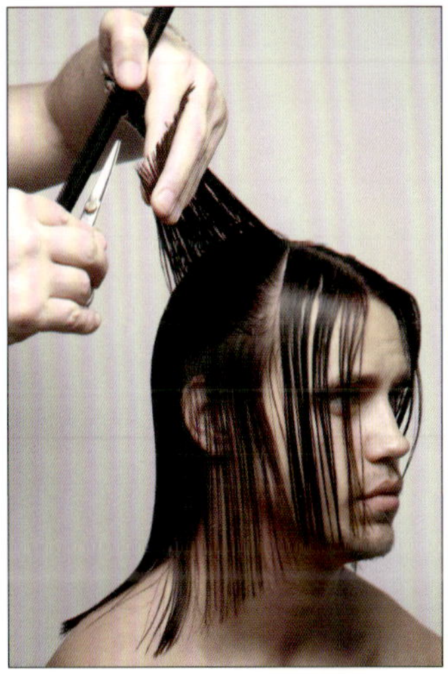

11 Wedge-shaped sections are taken from the profile line to the hairline at the sides and front of the head. Continue to follow the curve of the head.

12 Repeat the same process on the other side of the head. The sectioning pattern used remains the same. Cross-check the balance.

13 The perimeter can now be personalised by point cutting into the baseline, this will soften the edge and eliminate any excess weight.

14 For the finish, use an appropriate styling product and distribute evenly through the hair.

15 Using a hairdryer, the hair can either be power dried for maximum texture and separation, or, if a smoother finish is required, blow dry with a nozzle attachment on the hairdryer and use a metallic round brush.

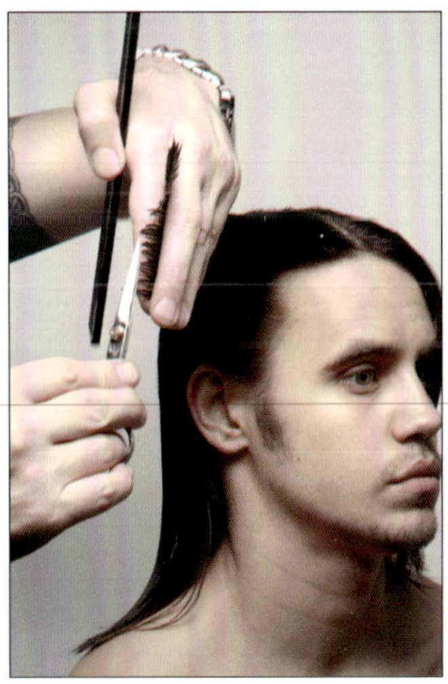

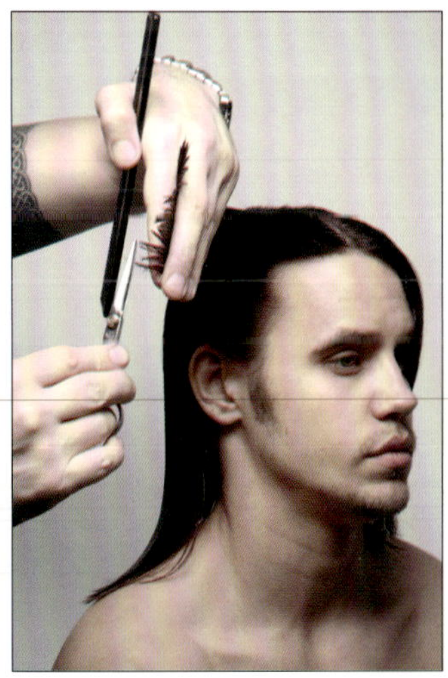

16 Starting at the back of the head, blow dry working around the head in halo-shaped sections.

17 Apply a finishing product to the hair. If the layers are short within the cut, work through a hair glaze and apply with the fingers to accentuate texture and separation in the finish.

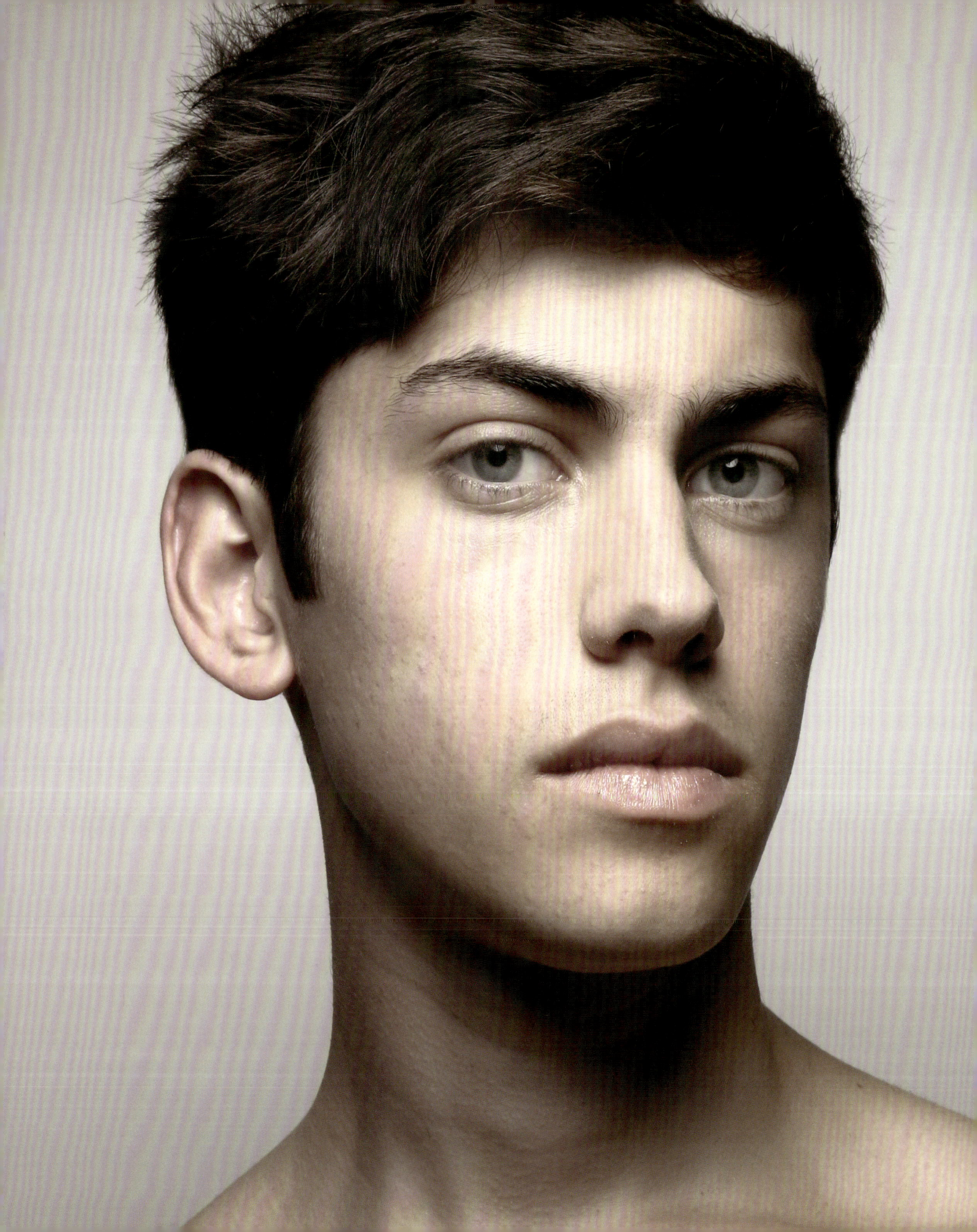

Square Graduation

The square graduation haircut is a truly versatile shape which looks equally as good on a man or woman. To create this shape, begin by working in vertical sections from beneath a horseshoe section by elevating out at a 45 degree angle, and progress around the head. Length is maintained through the top sections from the crown towards the front. This short layered shape can be blunt cut for a classic finish or point cut and chipped into to promote texture and separation.

When required, softness around the ear and nape area gives the woman's version more versatility, while a closer outline presents a masculine feel to the man's version.

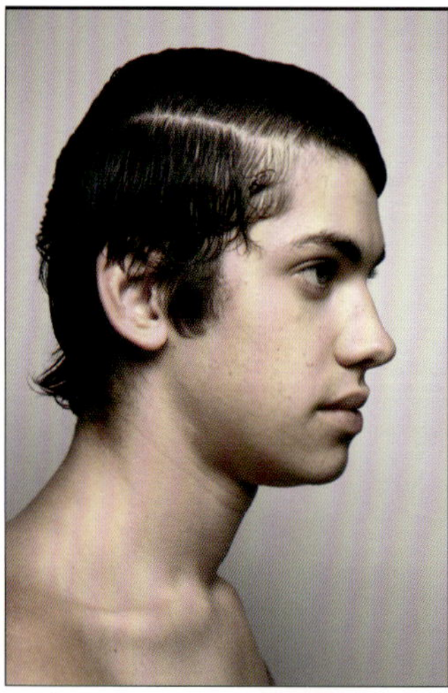
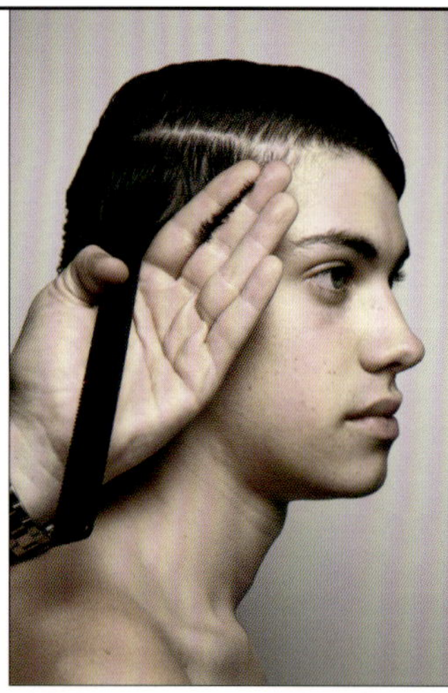
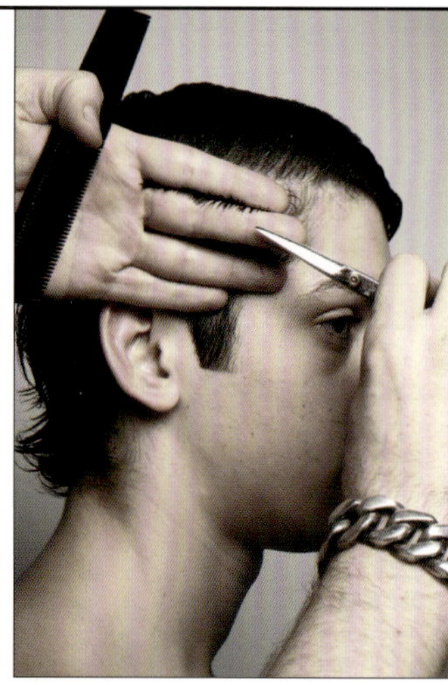
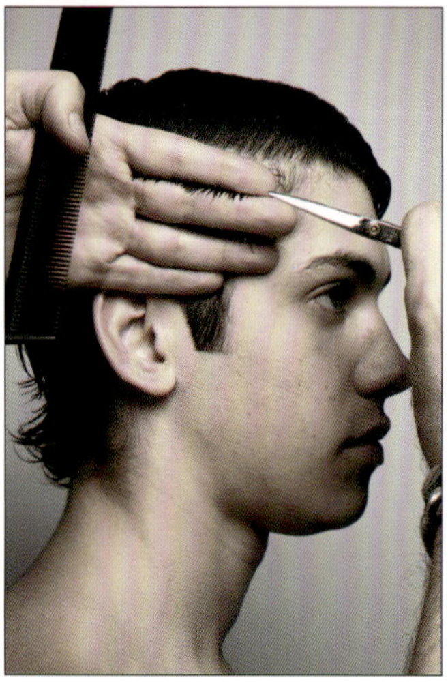
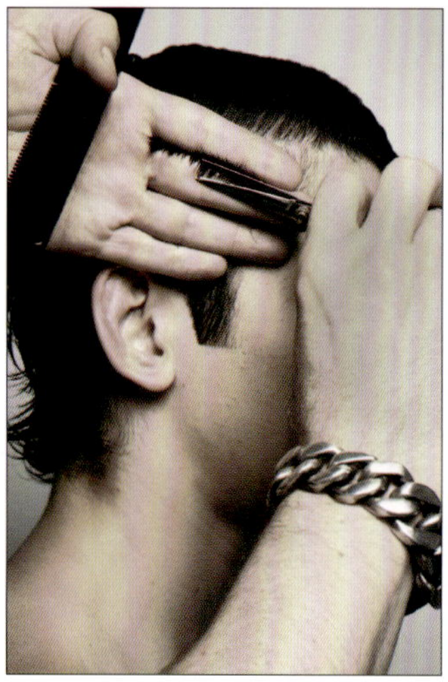
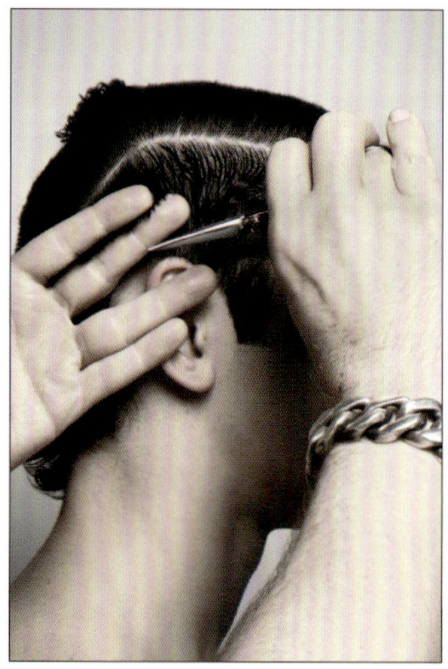
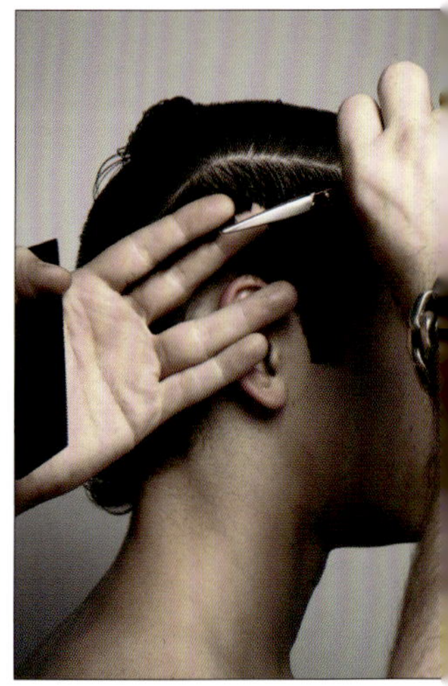

1 For the cut, after shampooing and conditioning, the hair is parted using a horseshoe section which runs from the recession area at the temples, and through the occipital bone at the centre back of the head. Section off the remaining hair on top of the head.

2 With the head in an upright position, on the side of the head at the front hairline, take a vertical section from the horseshoe parting down to the hairline just in front of the ear. Pull out at 45 degrees and determine the length, depending on the required finish, this technique could be blunt or point cut.

3 With the first section in place, this now becomes the guideline for each side of the haircut. Continue working in vertical sections using the pre-cut length as a guide on the side of the head. Work as far as the radial section and then cross-check by pulling out horizontal sections.

4 Repeat the exact same process on the other side of the head and then cross-check the balance on both sides of the head.

5 At the centre back take a vertical section from the horseshoe parting down to the hairline at the nape. Pull this section out at 45 degrees and cut the line from the occipital bone to the nape – this section becomes the guide for the back.

6 From the centre back continue working on the right hand side of the head. Take vertical sections around the back of the head out to behind the ear and connect into the side of the haircut. Repeat this procedure on the back left hand side, then cross-check the entire back section by taking horizontal sections, ensuring a smooth connection between the sides and the back.

7 The perimeter is then put in place at the back and sides of the head. Comb all the hair from the horseshoe parting down to the natural fall. Elevate out and point cut if a soft edge is required, or for a stronger outline work through the comb.

8 With the radial section still in place, from the crown take a vertical section down the centre back of the head and pull out at 45 degrees and make a connection from the crown to the occipital bone. On the right hand side of the head continue working around the back of the head and finish at the radial parting then repeat the same process on the left side. Check the entire back section by pulling out horizontal sections to cross-check.

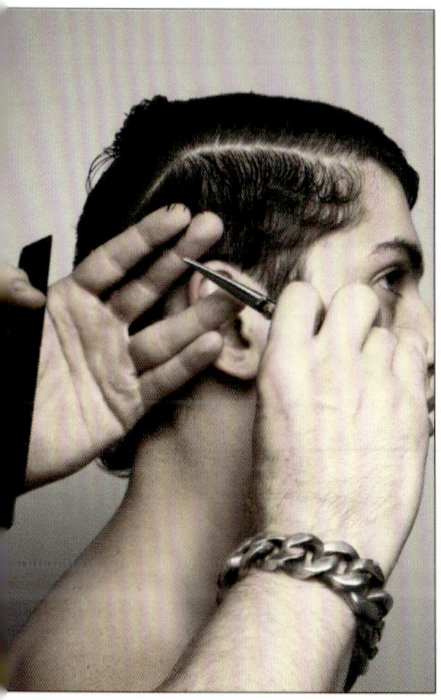
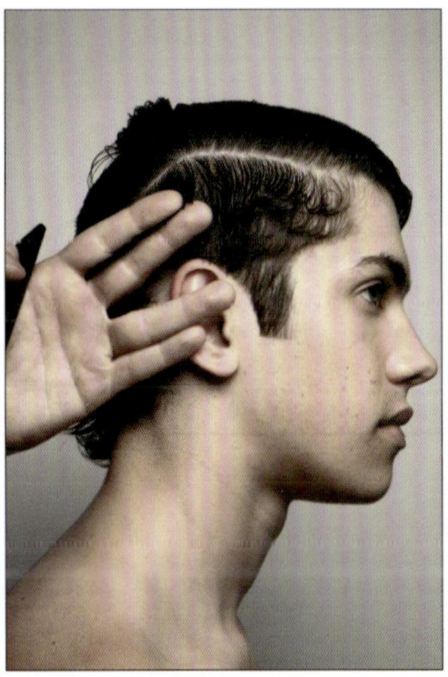
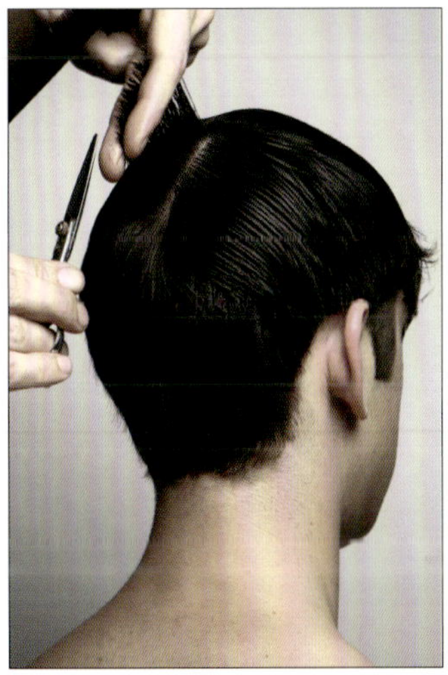
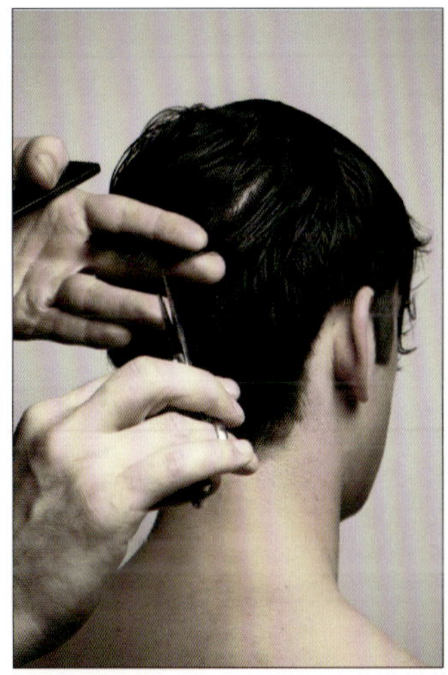

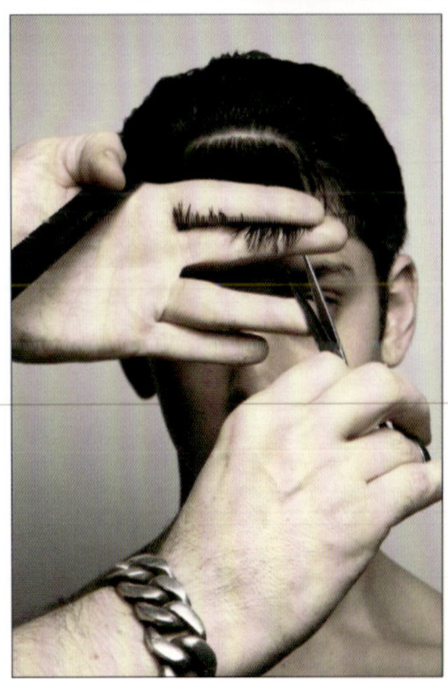
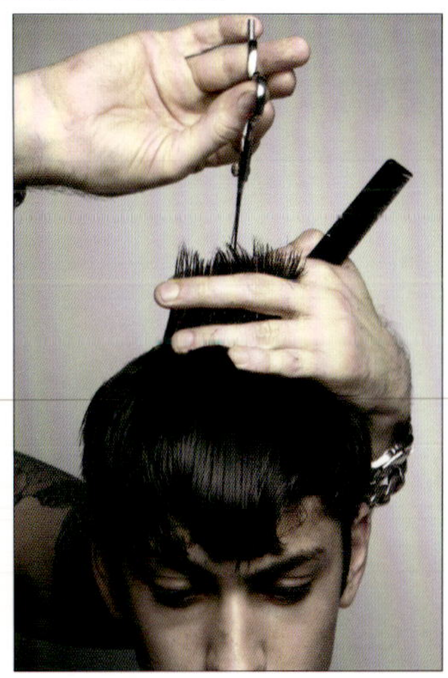

9 At the crown take a section from across the radial parting that incorporates the guide line, and pull up to 90 degrees. Cut following the guide.

10 Connect the back of the cut to the top by working from the crown down towards the front hairline, taking sections perpendicular to the sides of the head and pulling up to 90 degrees.

11 The perimeter through the front is then cut and connected into the sides. Cross-check the balance.

12 At the horseshoe section there may appear to be a slight disconnection; this area can be rounded off thus eliminating any excess weight build-up.

13 After cross-checking the haircut is complete.

14 For the finish, use an appropriate styling product and distribute evenly throughout the hair.

15 Depending on the finish required, the hair can either be power dried by using the fingers or blow dried with your choice of brush.

16 Once the hair is dried, the haircut can be personalised as required. Finally apply a finishing product to the hair to give maximum texture and separation.

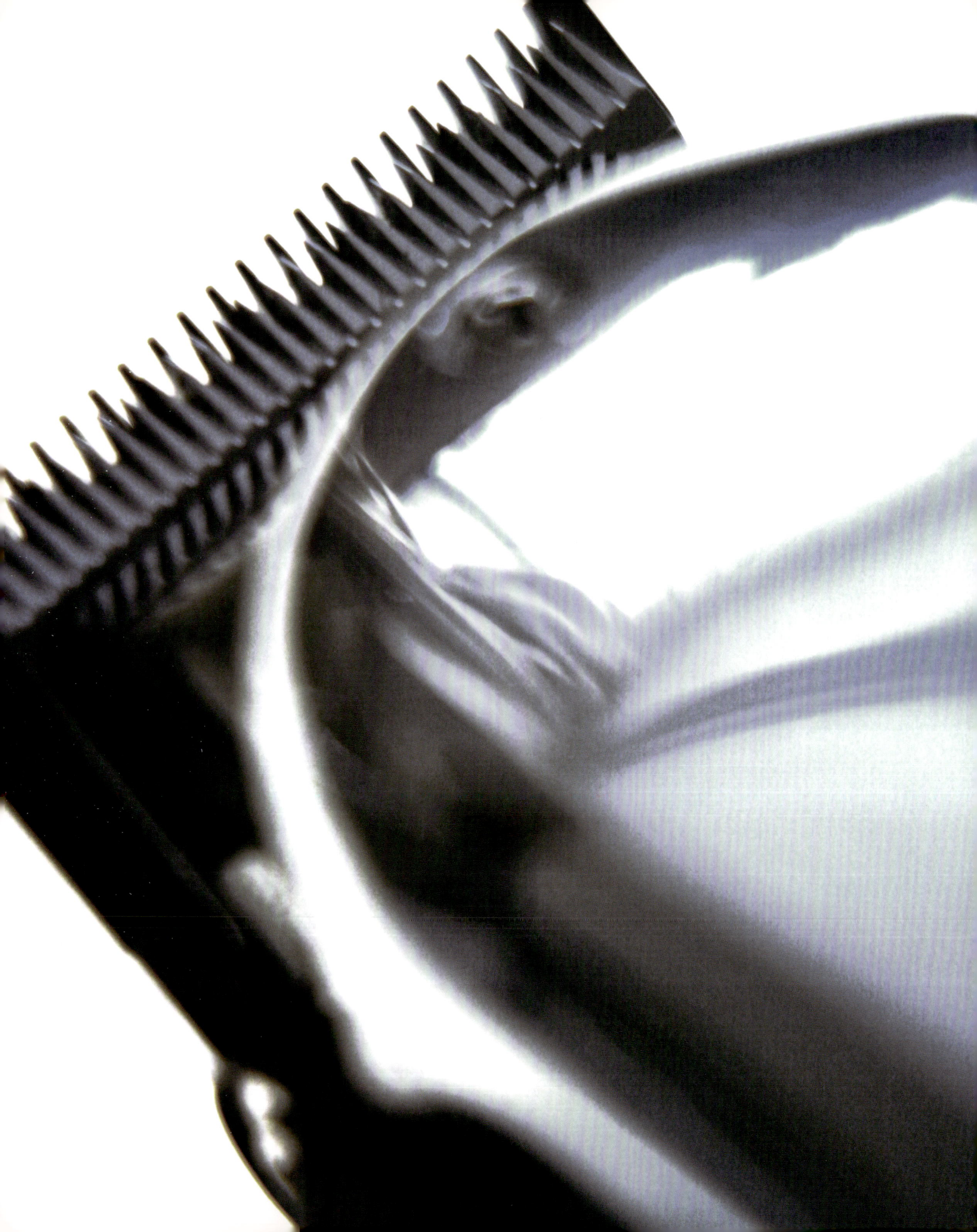

Scissor-over-Comb

This technique is often employed in men's hairdressing. It is used to cut hair very short, and follows the natural contour of the client's head. It is mainly used in the nape area and around the ears. If you use a barbering comb as well as a straight cutting comb, hair can be tapered very tightly into the hairline.

The scissor-over-comb technique can be used on both wet and dry hair; depending on hair texture and density, you may achieve a better result on dry hair. When working in the nape area remember to follow the natural growth pattern. Starting on the sides or at the back of the head, on the hairline, place the back of the comb on the head. The angle of the comb, always underneath the scissors, should be parallel to the head. The comb is always moved up, out and away from the head so as to avoid any harsh lines in the haircut.

Holding the scissors with the thumb and third finger, opening and closing the top blade with the back of the hand towards you, is the only way to cut the client's hair short enough in barbering. Progress up the head and cut a little hair at a time and always keep your scissor-over-comb work moving. Always take a guide line in the comb to the new length of hair to be cut – this is sometimes called a travelling guide. Connect the scissor-over-comb work to the graduation or weight line in the haircut.

Clipper work

Electric clippers are an essential piece of equipment in barbering and are available in a range of sizes. Clippers need to be kept clean and well maintained: the blades should be oiled regularly and be free from hair. If, during use, the clippers are pulling on the hair, try re-adjusting and cleaning the blades. Always replace the guard on the blade when the clippers are not in use.

The blades can easily be adjusted, normally by flicking a lever on the side of the clipper. The setting will vary between 1/20mm for the closest to 3mm for the greatest length in the cut. Clipper guards may also be used to vary the length of a haircut; the sizes used are 1, 2, 3 and 4 (Guard No.1 cuts the shortest, while No.4 gives the longest length). When using clippers on a client with a guard attachment, the guard will follow the shape of the head and follow the natural contour of the head as it moves over the scalp. So if the client has an uneven head shape then the haircut will also be uneven. This is sometimes why a scissor-over-comb technique takes preference as a means of cutting hair.

Colour

Colour Technique

Colour is made up from the spectrum of light, which has seven wavelengths of colour. These colours can be seen in a rainbow: red, orange, yellow, green, blue, indigo and violet. When light hits an object, some of the wavelengths are absorbed and some are reflected. Both these elements give the object its colour.

Primary Colours

The three primary colours are red, blue and yellow. From these three colours all other colours can be made. If all three primary colours were mixed together, this would give us black.

Secondary Colours

The three secondary colours are orange, violet and green. These colours can be achieved by mixing together true primary colours in the following way:

red + yellow = orange blue + red = violet yellow + blue = green

In hairdressing, a basic understanding of these principles can be used to select and apply colour in the best way for our clients. Colour has an enormous effect on all of us, be it physical, emotional or mental. We use light and colour every day. As colour is derived from light of varying wavelengths, and light is essential for all life, where would we be without it?

Tertiary Colours

There are six tertiary colours, achieved by mixing a primary and a secondary colour together: red mixed with violet, violet mixed with blue, blue mixed with green, green mixed with yellow, yellow mixed with orange and orange mixed with red.

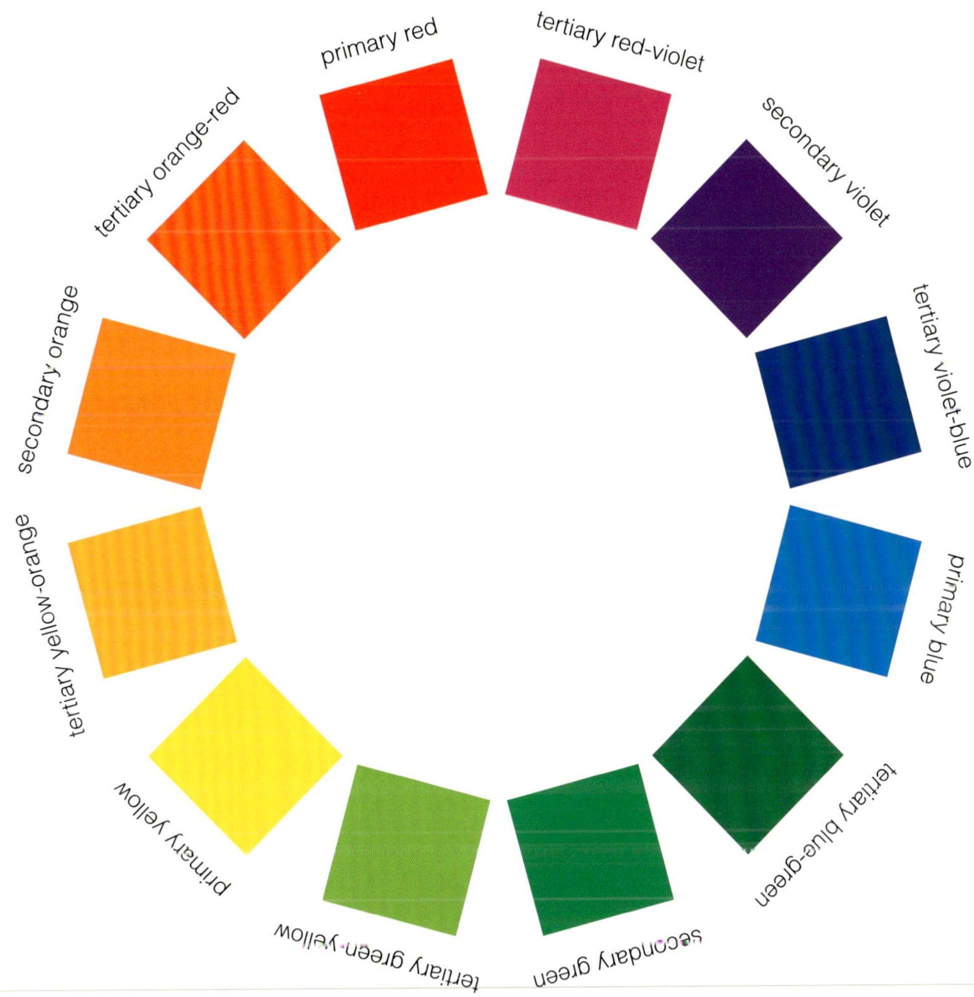

Complementary Colours

Complementary colours sit opposite each other on the colour wheel. For example, yellow and violet are complementary colours; orange is complimentary to blue and red is complementary to green. When complementary colours are placed side by side they appear brighter. It is important to have a balance of electric & cool, and magnetic & warm colours present in our lives, as they are good for our well-being.

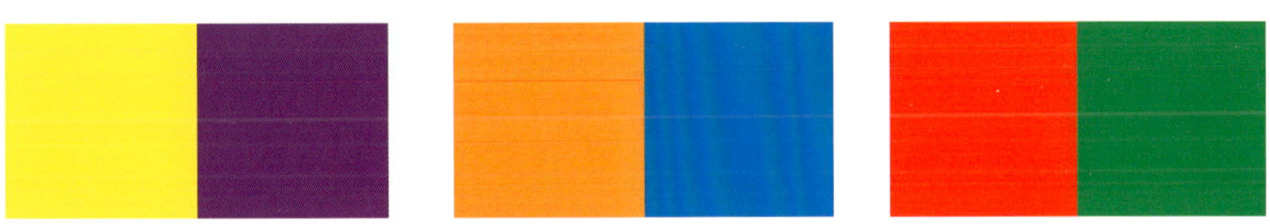

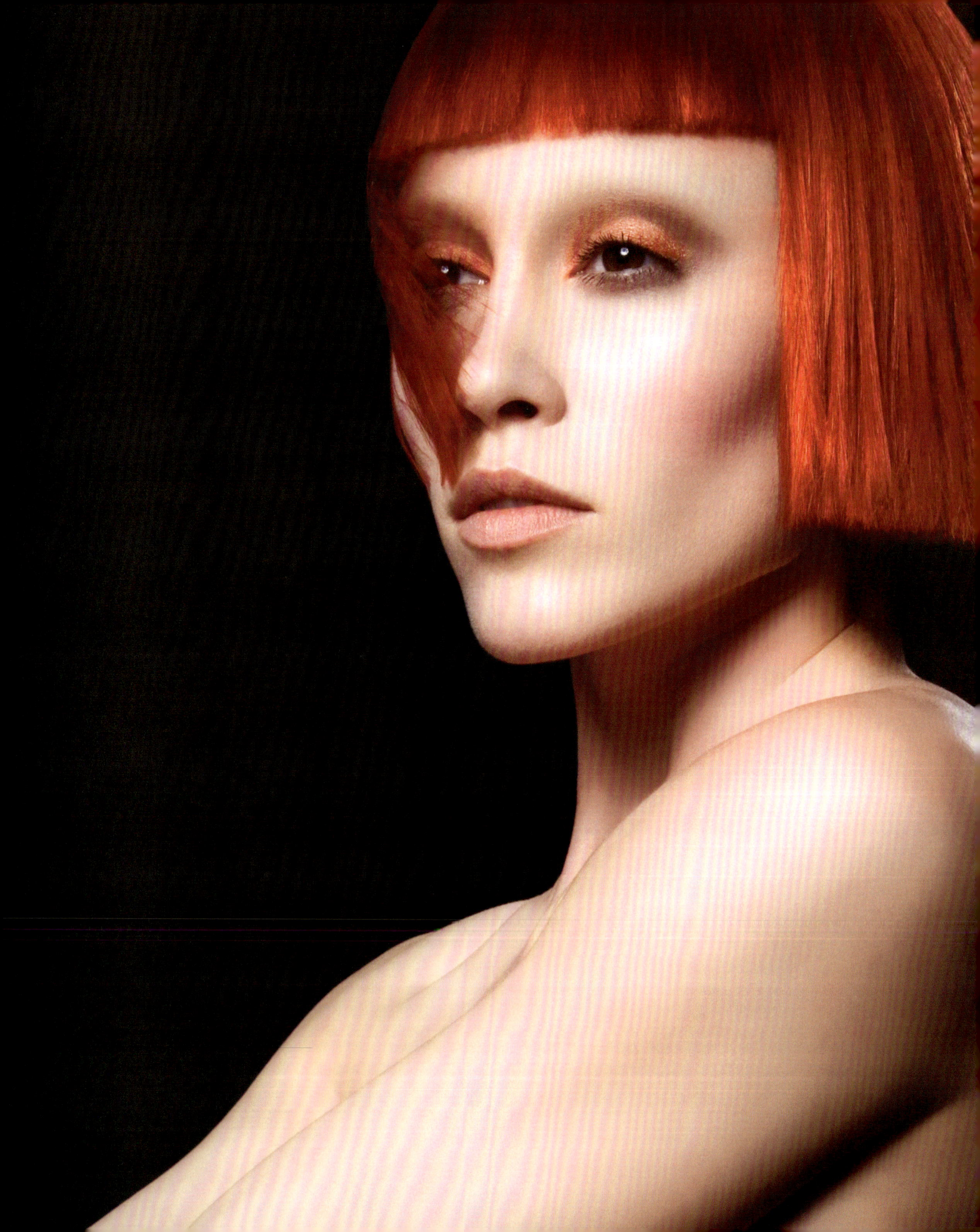

Hair Colour

The colour of human hair is divided into two areas: depth and tone.

Depth	Tone
10 – Lightest Blonde	/0 – Natural
9 – Very Light Blonde	/1 – Ash
8 – Light Blonde	/2 – Cool Ash
7 – Medium Blonde	/3 – Honey Gold
6 – Dark Blonde	/4 – Red Gold
5 – Light Brown	/5 – Purple
4 – Medium Brown	/6 – Violet
3 – Dark Brown	/7 – Brunette
2 – Black	/8 – Pearl Ash
1 – Intense Black	/9 – Soft Ash

For example, 7/03 would be Medium Natural Gold Blonde. The first number is the natural base. The numbers after the forward slash can be a combination of one or two tones.

Pigment

The natural depth of a client's hair tells us how light or dark the colour is. This also depends on the presence of pigment within the hair. Virgin hair has two types of pigment which are granular pigments and diffused pigments.

Granular pigments look like elongated molecules, which are black or brown in appearance; granular pigments are the easiest to remove when lightening hair.

Diffused pigments are yellow or red, and are smaller than granular pigments. As a result they can be a little more difficult to remove, because they are embedded deeper within the structure of the hair.

Everyone has both granular and diffused pigment present in their hair, but in various quantities. The less granular pigment there is in hair, the lighter it will be naturally; the more granular pigment present in the hair, the darker it will be. Having different combinations of pigment in our hair determines the hair colour we have.

Client Colour Consultation

Choosing a colour for the client depends on several factors, particularly the client's age and lifestyle – younger clients may want fashion colours, older clients may want to disguise white hair. It is all about suitability.

Determine the client's natural hair colour and what, if any, is the percentage of white hair present. To find the client's natural base shade look at the root area around the occipital bone as this will give you an accurate assessment of natural depth. Depth means how light or dark a colour is, tone means how warm or cool the colour is; a primary tone is dominant, a secondary tone is weaker. Decide what the target shade is, what product will be used, and what, if any, strength developer will be used.

The client's skin tone is also very important when choosing to colour hair – try to keep a balance between the two. A light ash blonde may not work against a dark skin tone. As we age the skin tone fades, so blue black would make the skin tone look paler than it actually is, if applied to a client of a certain age.

Assess the natural texture of a client's hair: is it coarse or fine? Colour applied to fine hair tends to develop and achieve a result quicker than it does on coarse hair. This is because there are usually more cuticle layers on coarse hair so the product has to work harder to penetrate the cortex where colour is deposited.

Take into consideration the condition and porosity of your client's hair. In the case of porous hair, the ends and sometimes the mid-lengths of the hair usually absorb product rapidly. If hair is very porous the final result may be an uneven colour. Leaving your client's hair in excellent condition after a colour service is paramount. To solve the problem of porosity, a course of intense conditioning treatments should be recommended to prepare the hair for colour.

Before you start work on your client's hair decide on what product you will use. Work with the shade chart as a visual guide, so your client has an accurate idea and can agree on the product. Advise your client on how you will achieve the colour, how long it will last, how it will affect their hair, how to maintain the colour, how much it will cost, advise on suitability and after care. Be as realistic as possible during your consultation with your client. Again it is about suitability.

Finally, as with any consultation, listen and communicate; welcome your client and be professional and friendly; discuss what the best options are.

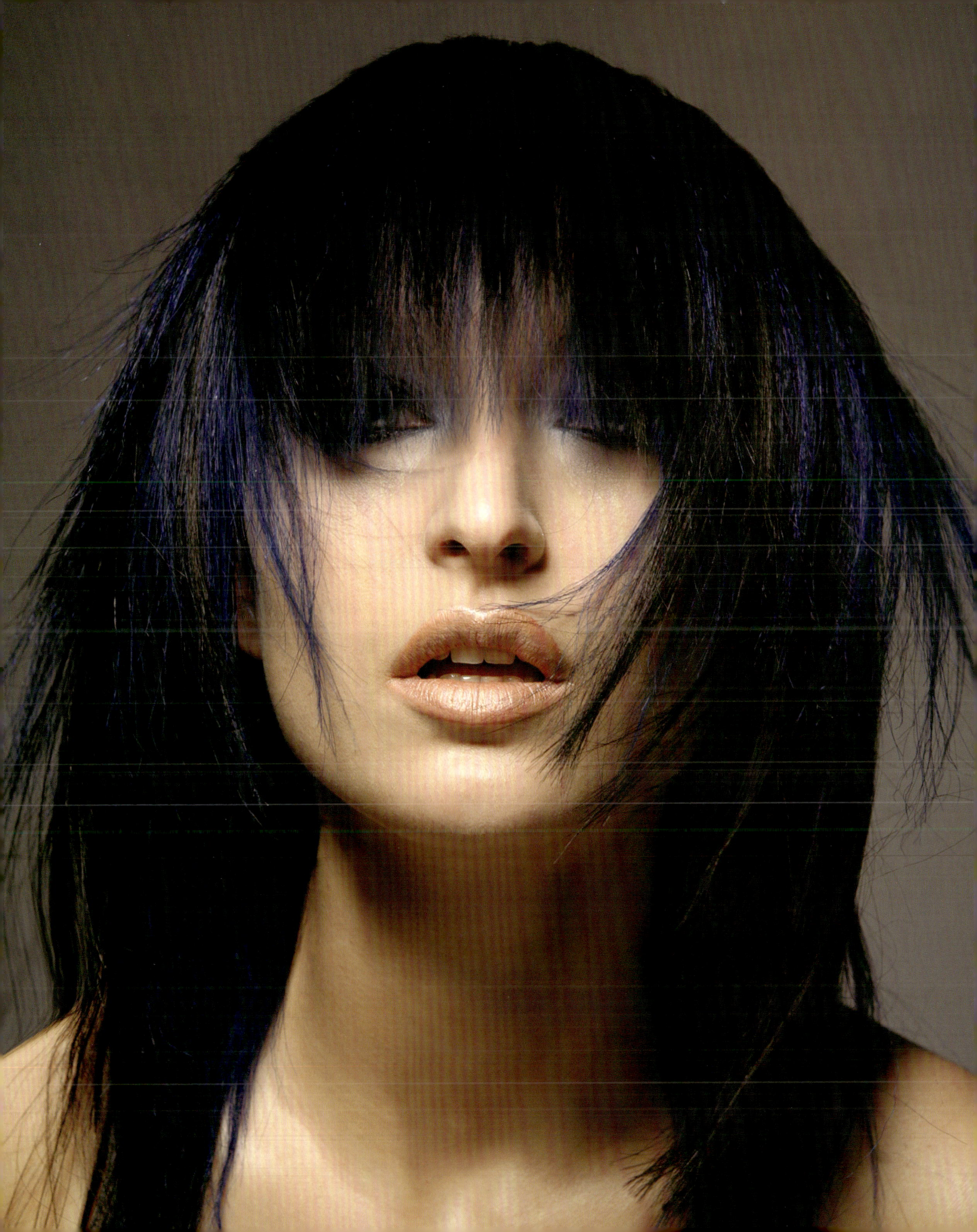

Temporary Colour

Temporary colours come in the form of mousse, colour enhancing shampoo, rinse, gel, cream and setting lotion and are usually applied to wet hair and dried into the hair, so no development time is required. These products will not permanently change the natural base of hair. Temporary colour molecules lie on the surface of the cuticle – they do not penetrate the hair shaft. The colour pigments in these products are fairly large and can be vegetable-based.

Temporary colour is often a way to introduce clients to colour and can also be used to produce fashion effects and bright crazy colour effects on pre-lightened or white hair. Yellow sometimes found on white hair can be neutralised or subtly toned. Temporary hair colour products are available in a wide range of shades. The product can be removed with one to six shampoos, although this will depend on the porosity of the client's hair. Hair cannot be lightened with a temporary colour and no skin test will be required. Sometimes a temporary colour can be applied to refresh a permanent colour in between salon visits. Temporary colour is applied directly onto the hair with no developer. Make sure of even distribution when applying it.

Semi-permanent Colour

Semi-permanent colours usually come in liquid form and no mixing is required. They are available in many shades and, depending on the porosity of the client's hair, normally last around six to eight shampoos. Semi-permanent colour lasts longer than temporary colour. The product is applied directly onto wet hair and no developer is required. The development time will depend on the individual manufacturer's instructions. Semi-permanent colour molecules are a combination of large and small in size, and lie partly in the cortex and partly between the cuticle and cortex.

A semi-permanent colour can be used as an alternative if a client is allergic to permanent colour, and it's also a way of introducing colour to clients who are generally shy of colour. Semi-permanent colour is an ideal way of maintaining the condition and vitality of the client's hair – it gives great shine to hair. Semi-permanent colour contains good quality conditioning ingredients and no ammonia or hydrogen peroxide, so there is no re-growth except if applied onto very porous or pre-lightened hair.

These products can be used as part of colour correction and pre-pigmentation work; they can also be used to refresh a permanent colour. Semi-permanent colours do not cover large percentages of white hair; however they can be used to blend and mask white hair. A skin test may be needed. This tends to vary with each manufacturer – again check instructions for use.

Quasi Colour

Quasi colour is also known as tone on tone hair colour, or a longer lasting semi-permanent colour. Quasi colour comes in the form of a cream or gel and can be applied with an applicator bottle as the consistency is fairly loose and can run. A quasi is mixed with a developer containing hydrogen peroxide, at a low strength between 1.9% and 4%. A quasi can be applied to wet or dry hair, and development times vary – again refer to manufacturers' instructions.

The molecules in a quasi are small to medium in size. They pass through the cuticle and are deposited into the cortex. Quasi colours usually last for about 10 to 20 shampoos; this depends on the porosity of your client's hair. Some re-growth will occur. They can add a beautiful shine and improve the condition of your client's hair. The client will be required to have a skin test before the service is carried out. Quasi colours come in a wide range of shades and can be used to blend and mask white hair.

Permanent Colour

Permanent hair colour usually comes in the form of cream or gel. The process of permanently colouring hair is known as tinting. The product is applied to dry hair and is mixed with hydrogen peroxide. Mixing is usually one part tint to two parts hydrogen peroxide – refer to manufacturers' instructions for correct amounts and strengths. The tint contains a substance known as para dye which is alkaline. Para dye molecules are small in size enabling them to pass through the cuticle to penetrate the cortex. Development begins as the para dye molecules mix with oxygen from the hydrogen peroxide. The molecules swell in size and remain trapped inside the cortex: this process is an oxidation reaction called polymerisation.

Once the colour has been applied to the hair, heat can be used if recommended by the manufacturer. This will speed up the development process. When developed, these molecules are permanently fixed inside the cortex. After development, emulsify, shampoo and condition the hair with pH-balanced products. The cuticle will then close down. Permanent colour can lighten up to three shades above the natural base and will darken below the natural base. A re-growth will occur with permanent colour. Tone can be added and it will cover any percentage of white hair. Before carrying out a permanent colouring service (24–48 hours ahead), a skin test will be needed to guard against allergic reaction.

Temporary Colour

Temporary colour is a direct dye as no mixing or skin test is required. These colours can be used directly from the bottle or applicator. Large colour molecules coat the outside of the cuticle. The duration is usually one shampoo, depending on the porosity of the hair.

Semi-permanent Colour

Semi-permanent colour is a direct dye as no mixing is required. It adds tone or darkens hair. Small colour pigments penetrate just slightly under the cuticle. The duration lasts to around six to eight shampoos depending on the porosity of the hair.

Quasi Colour

This is an indirect dye, as the product must be mixed with a developer to activate it. Small molecules pass through the cuticle and enter the edge of the cortex; the pigments swell and bind together and become fixed into the hair shaft. Skin test required.

Permanent Colour

Is an indirect dye, as the product is mixed with a developer. Some colour pigments pass through the cuticle and enter deep inside the cortex. The pigments swell and join together and are permanently fixed in the cortex. Skin test required.

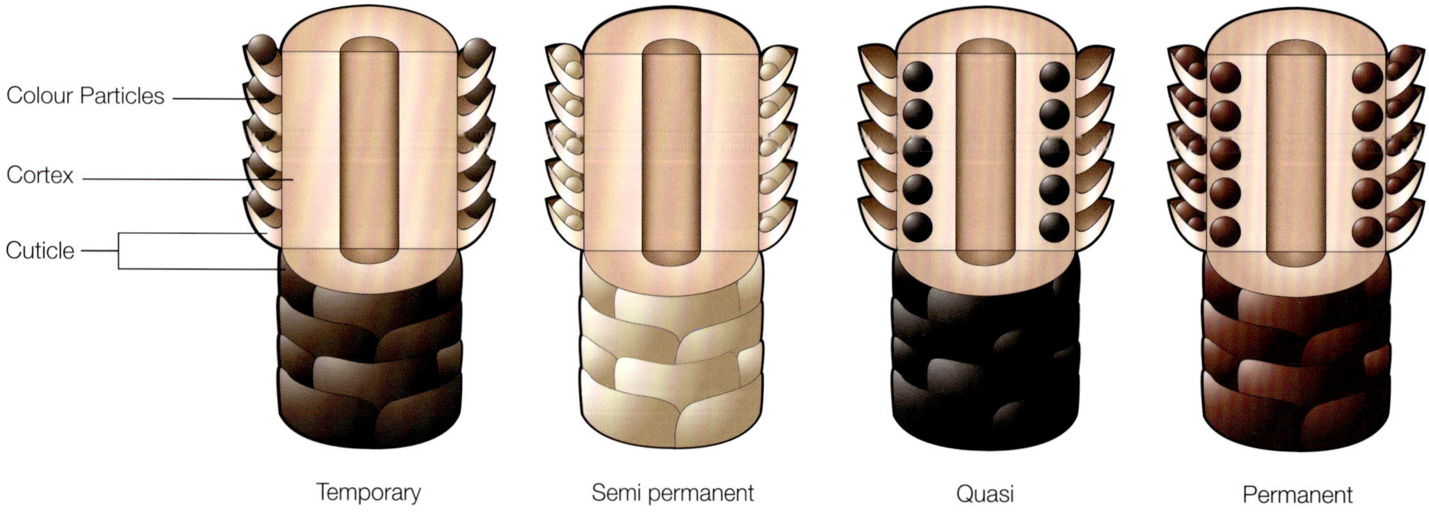

Hydrogen Peroxide

Hydrogen peroxide H202 is an activator mixed with quasi, permanent and bleaching products. It is usually available as a liquid or cream. Hydrogen peroxide comes in varying percentages or volumes. The most commonly used in hairdressing are:

3% or 10 volume
6% or 20 volume
9% or 30 volume
12% or 40 volume
18% or 60 volume

When hydrogen peroxide is mixed with colouring products oxygen is released. The higher the percentage or volume of hydrogen peroxide used, the more oxygen is released, giving higher lift in the colouring process. The lower the percentage or volume of hydrogen peroxide used, the lower the depth of colour is achieved. Different strengths of hydrogen peroxide produce different results. Depending on the amount of lift required, the following is a guide:

6% or 20 volume will give one level of lift
9% or 30 volume will give two to three levels of lift
12% or 40 volume will give three to four levels of lift

6% or 20 volume, when mixed with permanent colour products, will give coverage of white hair; it will darken hair and maintain the same colour as the client's natural base; it will also lighten up to one level when used on other base shade colours of hair.

Hydrogen peroxide will lose its strength if it is not stored properly. Caps should be screwed on tightly and containers placed in a cool dark place after use. Always follow the manufacturer's instructions.

Pre-Pigmentation

Pre-pigmentation is a process of adding colour pigment to hair. This is carried out because pigment may have been lost, removed or may never have been present. Pre-pigmentation is a way of ensuring that the final colour has the correct depth, tone and a durable colour result. It is advisable to pre-pigment when going two levels darker or lower as pre-pigmentation prevents fading on very porous hair. Think about the target shade before choosing the pre-pigment shade. If you want a cool target shade avoid using pigmentation with too much warmth.

This technique is usually used in colour correction. If returning a client's pre-lightened hair to its natural base, pre-pigmentation must be carried out or the resulting hair tone will be ash (or green) if permanent colouration is applied. Pre-pigmentation is a technique used to fill in the loss of red, orange and yellow pigment on pre-lightened porous hair. There are many techniques used to pre-pigment. For example, using your target shade, apply a temporary or semi-permanent colour to the hair. Allow to develop and remove any excess. Then apply permanent colour, with developer one shade lighter than your target shade, on top of the previous colour – and develop. Again follow the manufacturer's instructions according to the brand used.

Safe Colouring

Before applying any colour products, always follow the manufacturer's instructions. It is important to store, use and dispose of all colouring products carefully. Follow the health and safety policies as directed by your salon.

After any skin test and/or colouring process, record all details of the service for future reference.

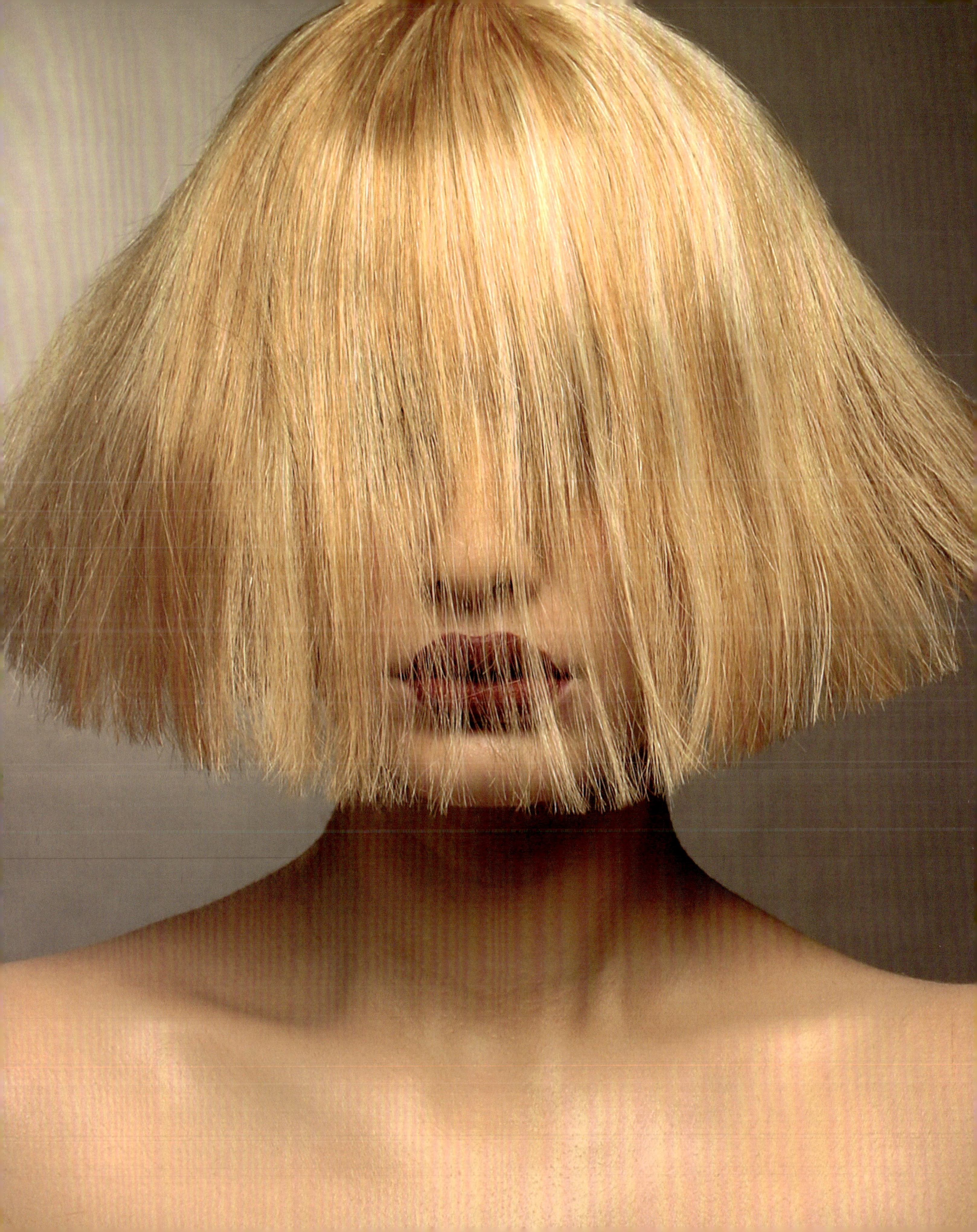

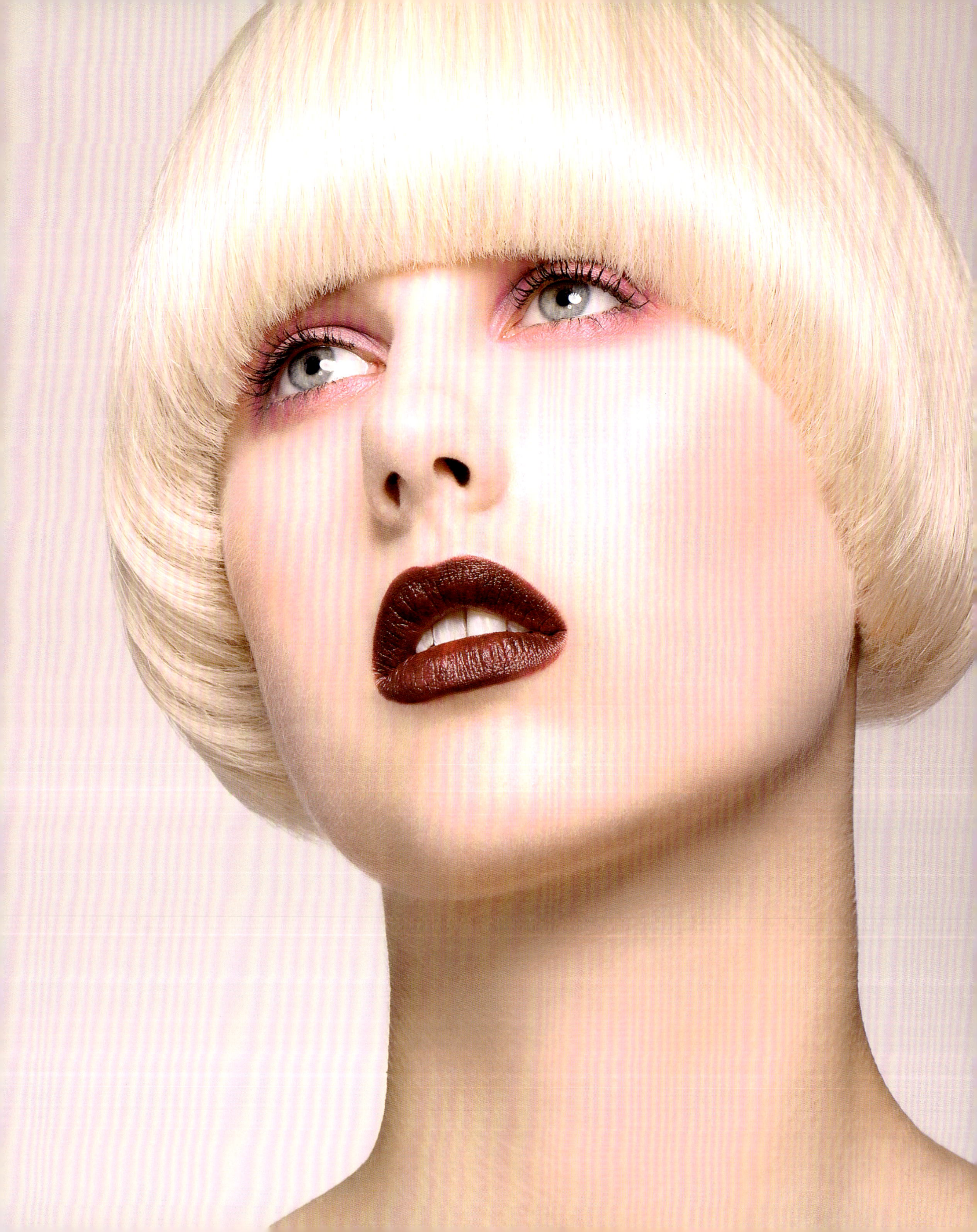

Bleach

A high lift tint will only give a certain level of lift. If further lift is needed then the hairdresser turns to bleach, which can achieve higher levels. The client's hair must be strong and in good condition to be able to go through the bleach or pre-lightening process. Bleach comes in two forms:

Powder is strong and used mainly for foil highlights and highlighting techniques. Hydrogen peroxide is added to powder bleach and mixed to a paste with a smooth consistency. Refer to manufacturers' instructions for quantities. If powder bleach is left exposed to air or heat it can dry out.

Emulsion is gentle and used for a full head on scalp application. This comes in the form of oil or gel. Emulsion bleaches are mixed with hydrogen peroxide; the strength used will depend on how dark the hair is and how much lift is required. Next a booster or activator is added to the mixture, usually a blue powder. This intensifies the strength of the emulsion. Again check the manufacturer's instructions for the recommended amounts.

Bleach is an alkaline product which works when added to hydrogen peroxide of varying strengths. Once the product has been mixed and is applied to the hair, the cuticle lifts and the product penetrates the cortex. Oxygen is released and the colour pigments in the hair shaft react and become oxymelanin or colourless. As this eumelanin process continues, the black and brown colour pigment present in hair, begins to disappear. Black pigment is the first to be lifted out, followed by brown; then pheomelanin pigments, which are red and yellow, are eliminated. Yellow is notoriously difficult to remove and is always the last one to be taken out, so some yellow may remain in the hair; this can be neutralised by adding a violet toner.

Bleach is applied to dry hair and can be used to achieve a variety of effects. When pre-lightening, use bleach to attain the level of lift required. When applying to a re-growth take care not to overlap hair that has previously been bleached, as the hair will become weaker and some breakage could occur. Checking the development of bleach is usually by observation. Bleach is a permanent colouration and re-growth will develop as the hair grows. When working with bleach try not to aim for too high a lift, as the danger of over-processing will result in the disintegration of the hair. Check the development process at regular intervals.

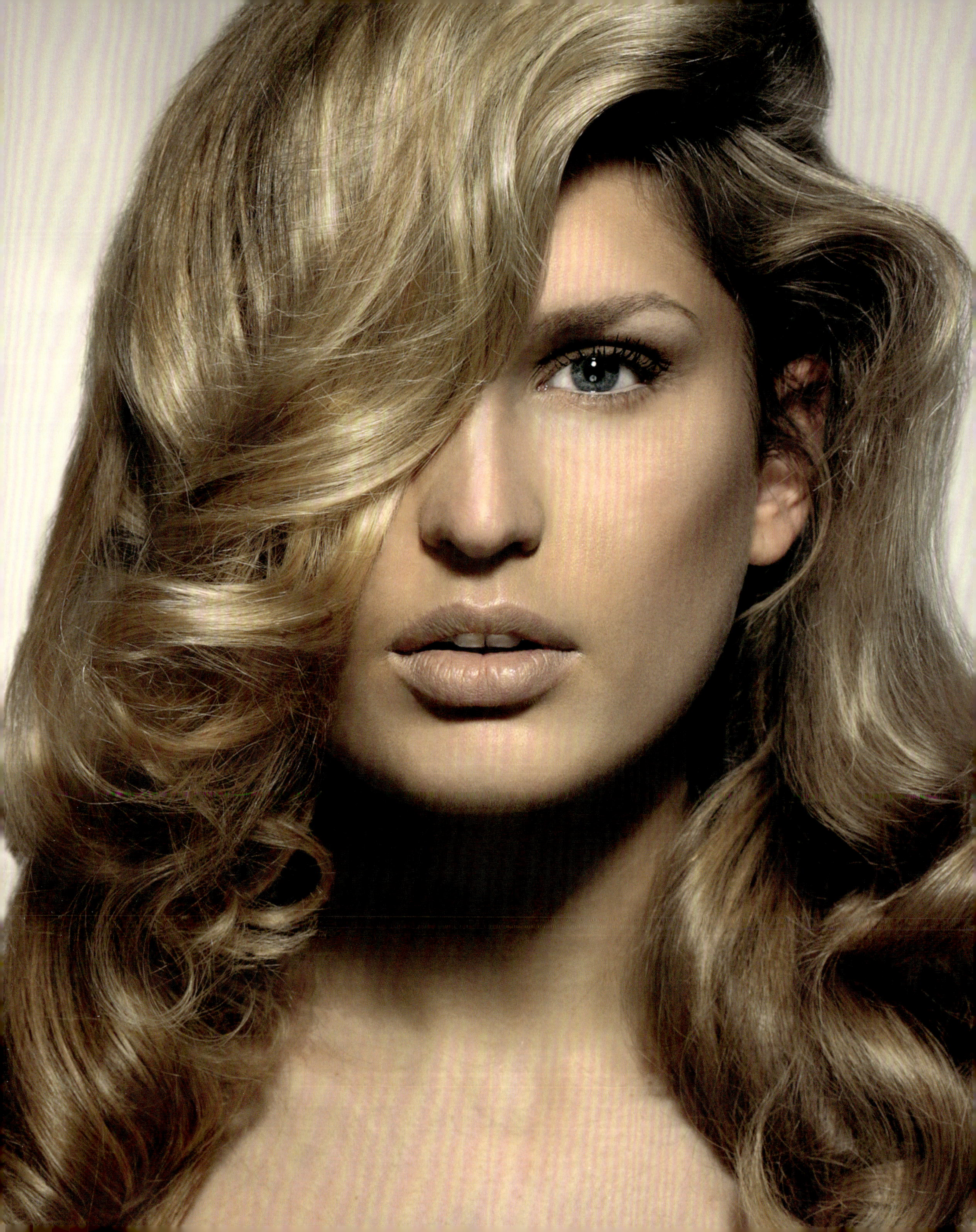

Highlights

Lightening products such as tint, high lift tint and bleach are often used for highlighting, especially where two levels of lift or more are required. The advantages of woven highlights are:

1. Colour can be applied close to the roots
2. More than one colour can be used on a set of highlights
3. Depending on result required tint and bleach can be applied to the same head
4. Colour can be applied directly to the area where required,
5. The application of colour is placed off scalp which helps if a client has a sensitive scalp or is allergic to tint.

Woven highlights often have variations in the placement procedure, for example, a 'T' section technique is applied where woven highlights are placed around the crown area, down along the parting and around the front hairline. This application forms a 'T' shape hence the name for this technique.

Another technique, Half Head Highlights are usually worked just above the occipital bone at the back of the head, then by progressing through the crown area and continuing along the top of the head towards the front hairline, then working down each side of the head and incorporating the hairline around the ears.

A Full Head Highlights application follows a sectioning pattern which will give the client a full head of woven highlights. A further application for woven highlights could be described as a fashion technique where placement of colour could be applied in a directional pattern to complement and personalise the client's hairstyle.

Foil is used for woven highlights, the width of foil usually comes as standard on a roll from the manufacturer. The roll of foil is usually housed in a dispenser and lengths of foil are torn off to a size which is workable to the length of the section of hair to be woven. Apart from silver, other colours of foil are available; if highlighting the client's hair with more than one colour, choose a coloured foil in conjunction with the tint being used. This method will give colour placement where needed and will help stop getting the application uneven in the running order of the various shades of colour being used.

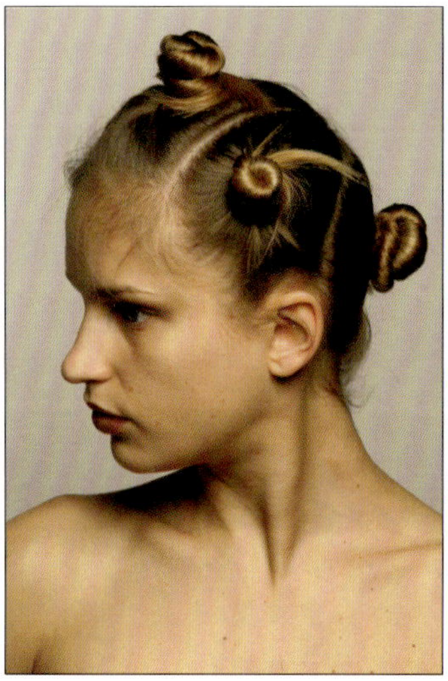

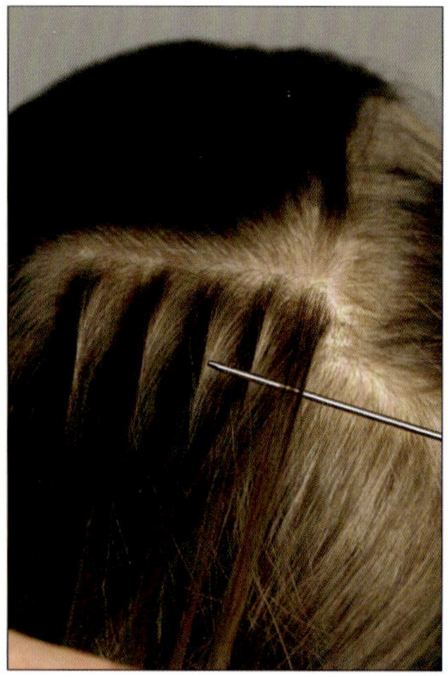

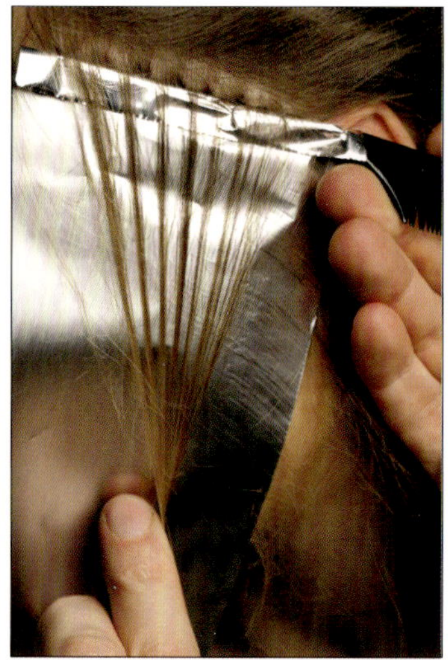

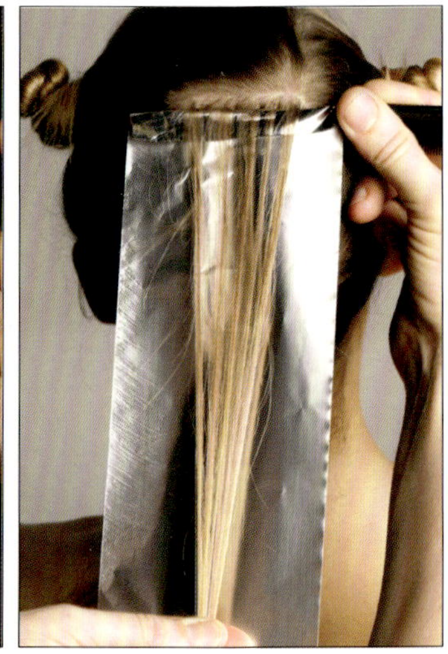

The basic principles of woven highlights are quite straight forward. Proceed by greeting your client and carry out a colour consultation. If it's a first time application for the client, advise on colour suitability, decide on how fine/thick the woven highlights will be? Start by examining the condition of the client's hair and scalp. Advise on after care and frequency of re-growth application.

The application of woven highlights usually depends on the technique being used. Techniques to take into consideration are 'T' section, Half Head, Full Head or Fashion techniques. If the client is returning to the salon for re-growth coverage and wants to maintain the previous application, simply follow the formula and information that is written on the client's record card.

1 After deciding on the technique, prepare the client and your equipment for highlighting. Divide the hair into sections, again the sections will depend on how the service is being carried out.

2 With a pin tail comb take a fine section and weave out close to the root area, place foil underneath the woven section and as close to the roots as possible.

3 Apply colour product directly onto the woven section. Begin at the root area and work the product onto mid-lengths and ends for a first time application or re-growth as required.

4 Seal the packet at the top and sides. If too much product is applied, it could leak out of the packet and onto the scalp or areas of hair not requiring colour and could leave a very undesirable patchy result.

5 Ensure that the woven out section underneath the packet is sectioned away before starting on the next section.

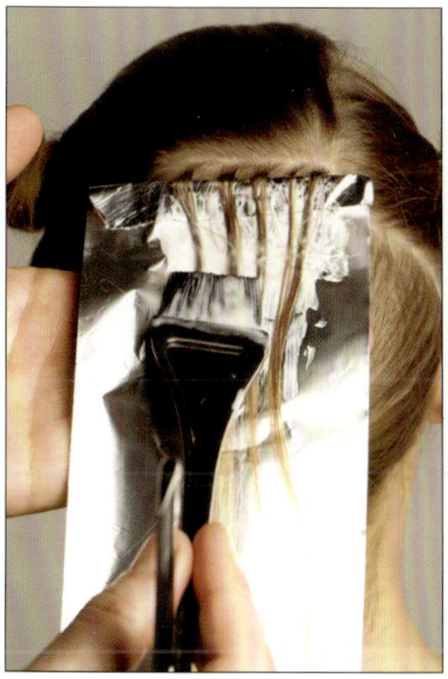
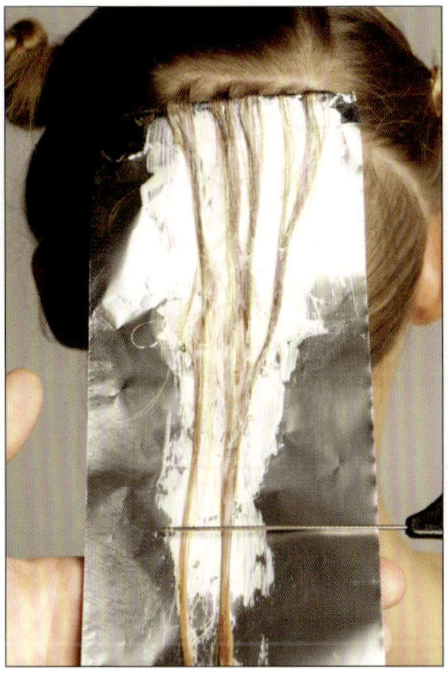
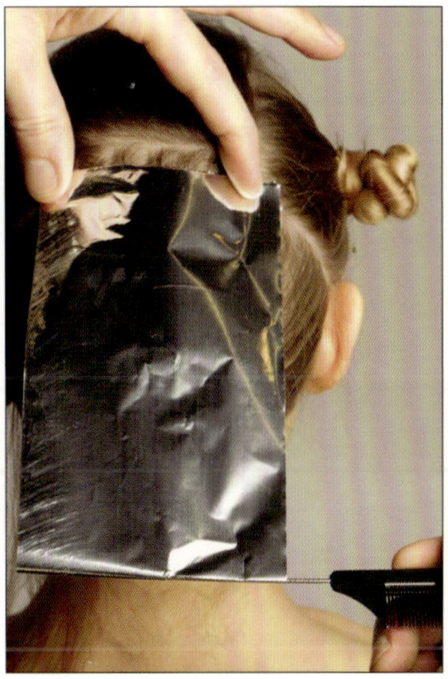
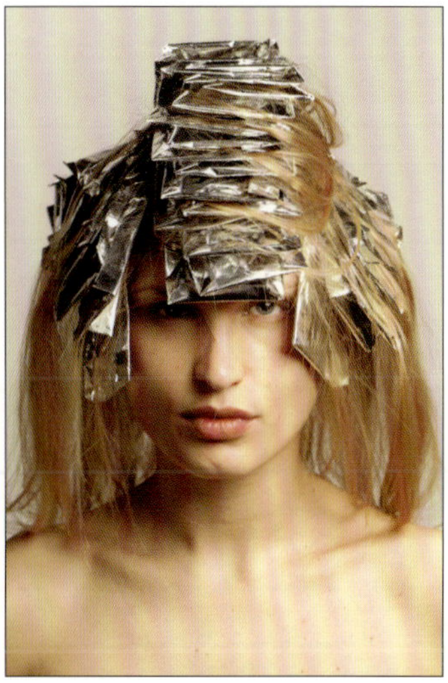

6 Highlighting can be a lengthy process especially when working on a full head application. When using bleach products, some of the highlights will have developed before all sections have been completed, check the development whilst progressing through the application, if some of the highlights have fully developed, open the foils and with cotton wool remove the product and apply antioxidant conditioner, this will stop further development and will result in an even shade of colour throughout.

7 If highlighting a client's hair and the process becomes time consuming you may have to mix a fresh bowl of product. This is done in order to keep consistency throughout as some products will lose their strength after a certain period of time. Development times of products may vary, check with the manufacturer's instructions. Once highlights have developed, remove foils, rinse, emulsify, shampoo and condition the hair.

8 Lowlights are applied in exactly the same way as highlights, the only difference being the choice of product. Lowlights can be recommended to clients who may require more depth or tone to their hair. Deeper, richer shades of brown, mahogany, red, gold and classic naturals are often used in lowlighting. Again more than one shade may be used on any individual client, do think about suitability when working within the client's natural base. The advantage of lowlights is that regrowth is less obvious and the method is an off scalp application. Clients with a low to medium percentage of white hair may prefer lowlights to blend with their natural base.

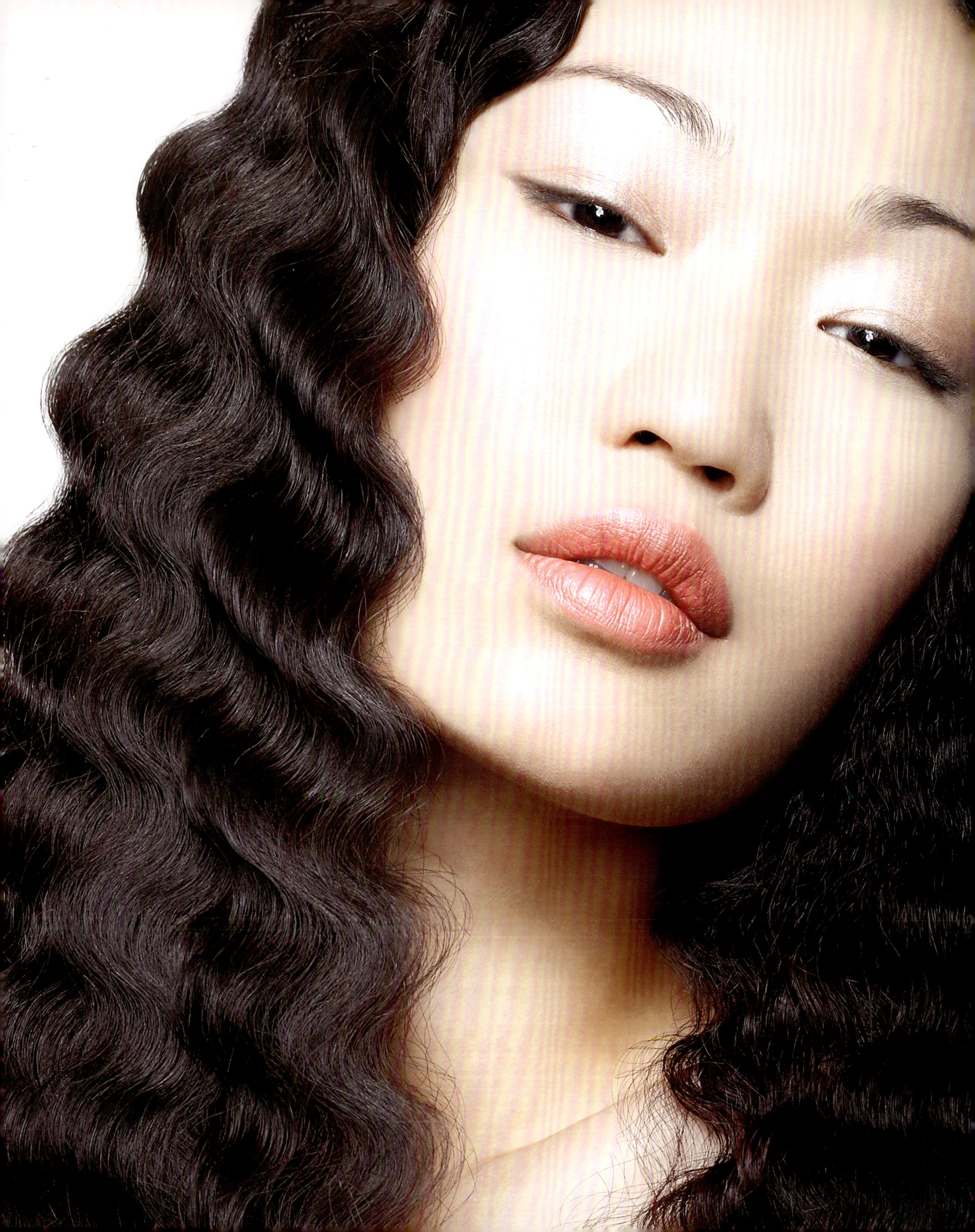

Permanent Wave

Perming is a technique used to describe curling or waving hair permanently. It is a chemical process that alters the structure of the hair. There are three stages of perming.

In the first stage, hair is softened by the perm solution. In the second stage it is moulded, taking the form of the rod or curler it is wrapped around. Thirdly, after development, the hair is permanently fixed into its new form by going through a process called neutralising.

When hair is permed, the chemical structure of the hair is altered. The disulphide bridges that give hair its strength are broken during the perming process, making the hair softer. This allows it to take the form of the size of curling rod used. When perm solution is applied to hair it passes through the cuticle and penetrates the cortex. Hydrogen in the lotion breaks the disulphide bridges and the keratin is now in beta keratin stretched form.

Not all the disulphide bridges need to be broken. If too many are, this may result in over-processing and will damage the hair. During the development process check the perm at regular intervals. After taking a test curl and seeing that the desired result has been reached, stop the softening process by rinsing away the perm solution with warm water.

Next, neutralise to re-form and harden the hair. New disulphide bridges are made as the hydrogen reacts with the oxygen in the neutralising agent. Oxidisation takes place and the keratin in the hair is now in a new alpha keratin, unstretched form. After completing the process, the hair has been permanently waved or curled. This will last until the perm grows out of the hair.

Permanent Wave Consultation

As with any consultation discuss the requirements of a perm with your client. Again, it is all about suitability – take hairstyle and life style into consideration. Are there any reasons why you would advise against your client having a perm? Are there any contraindications – is the hair or scalp in poor condition?

Never perm on hair that has been treated with products containing metallic salts: henna for example. Pregnant women should be advised against a chemical service, as pregnancy hormones have an effect on hair.

The degree of curl depends on the size of the rod used. A larger rod will give loose waves or a soft curl, as a smaller rod will give a tighter more defined curl. Hair length should also be taken into consideration when deciding on a perm.

What result will you achieve on the hair with a perm? Which is the best lotion to use? Will the perm be left to dry naturally or will it be set or blow dried? Again, think about what is realistic. What condition will the hair be left in after a perm and how will the client care for the perm at home?

As with all chemical services, before starting work on your client's hair, read and check manufacturers' instructions and record results for your reference.

Alkaline Perms

They have high alkalinity with a pH of usually around 9.5. The higher the pH of the perm solution, the more damaging it can be to the hair. Alkaline perm solution is very strong and will give a very defined curl. Ammonium thioglycollate is the main chemical in an alkaline perm solution. Alkaline perms are very long lasting and are used on resistant hair; they tend to process quickly and heat is not always required. The use of an alkaline perm on hair that has previously been chemically treated with bleach or high lift tint is not recommended. If hair is porous carry out the necessary tests.

Acid Perms

The main chemical in an acid perm is glyceryl monothioglycolate. Glyceryl monothioglycolate works by breaking the disulphide bridges between the polypeptide bonds in the keratin. This chemical contains no ammonia is not associated with the odour that alkaline perms have. Within the EU there is a downward trend towards the use of acid perms, the reason being glyceryl monothioglycolate usually reveals hypersensitivity to the chemical. If using this chemical hairdressers may develop dermatitis on their hands. Clients who are sensitive to glyceryl monothioglycolate may suffer dermatitis on the neck, scalp and ears. The chemical can remain active in hair and may cause dermatitis. To determine glyceryl monothioglycolate sensitization, carry out a skin test. Acid perms are a gentler alternative to alkaline perms and they produce a much softer curl. Activators are added to acid perm solution, acid perms rely upon heat to open up the cuticle to allow the perm solution to penetrate the cortex. During processing there are fewer bonds broken in the hair structure, which makes it an ideal choice to use on hair that is more fragile or chemically treated. The pH of an acid perm is usually around 6.5 which is close to the acid mantle of human hair. True acid perms have become less frequently manufactured – alkaline perm lotions are now more commonly used.

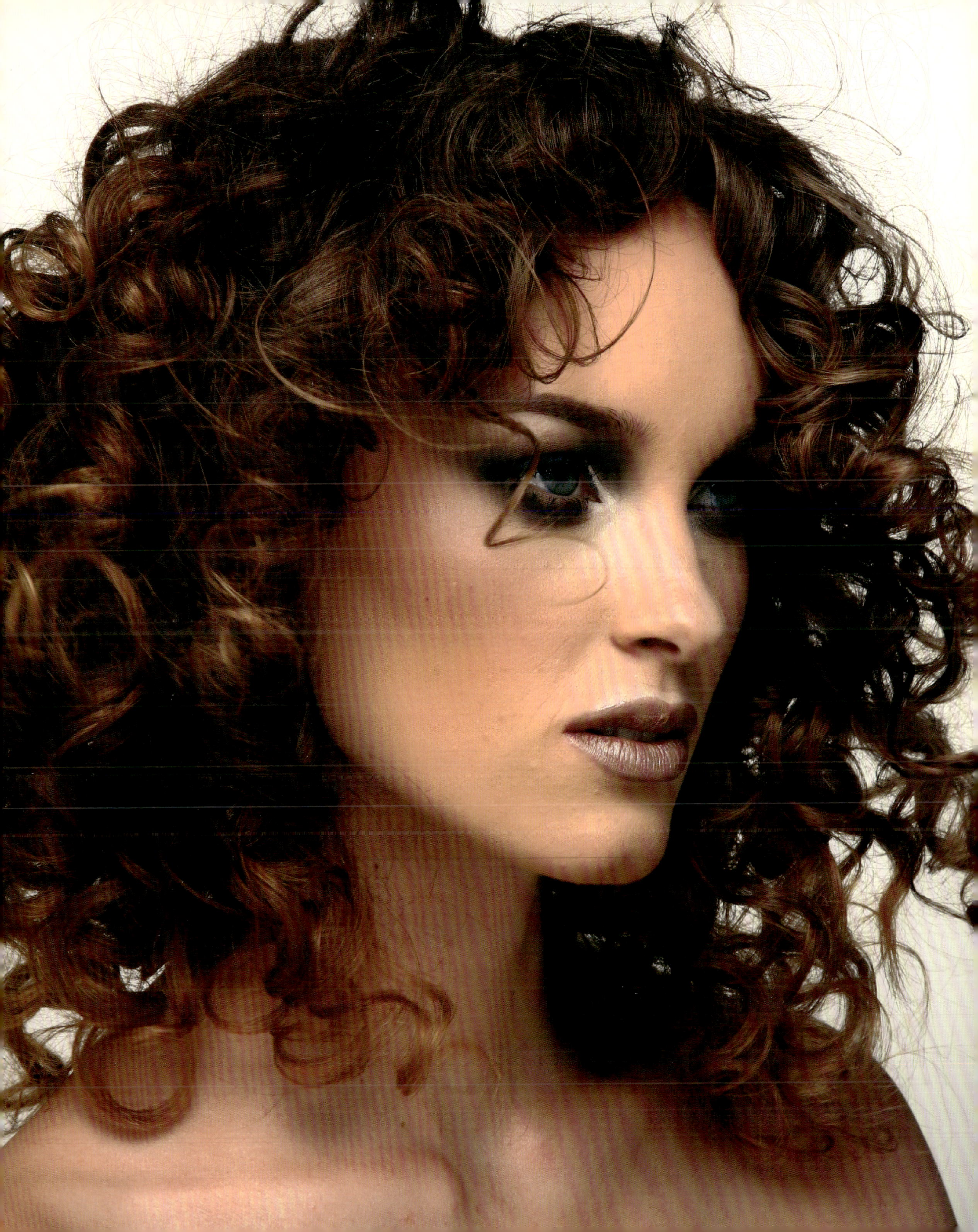

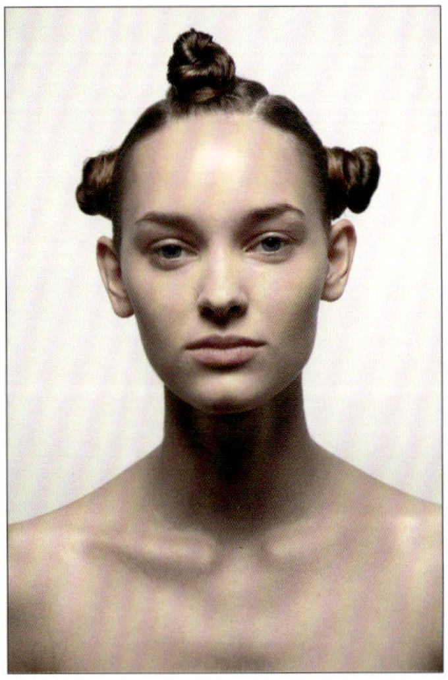

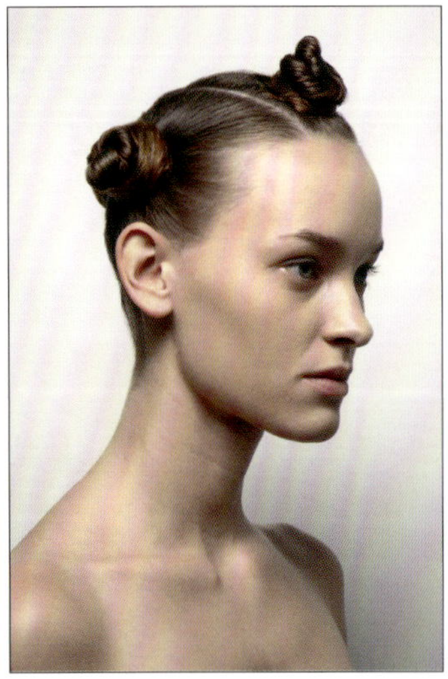

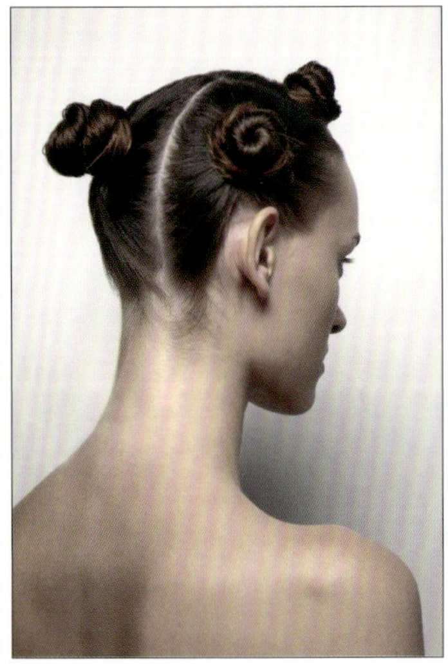

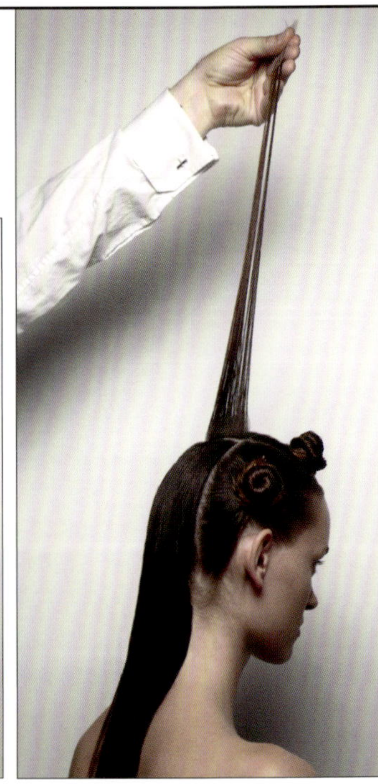

Perm Rods and End Papers

Perm rods are available in various sizes. If you use a large rod on your client's hair the result will be a soft curl or wave: alternatively if you use a small rod, this will result in a tighter more defined curl.

End papers are used in the winding process of perming. You tear them off from a pad of absorbent papers, and fold each individual end paper around a section of hair just before the hair is wound around a rod. End papers are designed to keep the ends of the hair straight, and prevent them from becoming hooked or buckled during the winding process.

Sectioning – The First Panel

Sectioning is carried out on hair that has been shampooed and towel dried; usually there is no need to condition the hair before a perm. There are various methods of taking sections for a perm. The following describes a classic wind.

The size of the section taken will depend on the size of rod you are working with, taking into consideration its length and circumference. The width of the section should be slightly narrower than the length of the rod; but it should be around the same depth as the circumference of the rod, to allow the rod to sit on top of its section.

With the client's head in an upright position, begin by parting the hair from the crown and take a radial section to behind the back of each ear. Then sub-divide by taking a central panel down the centre back of the head to the hair line in the nape. This section should be slightly narrower than the length of the rod being used. Continue the sub-section towards the front hair line.

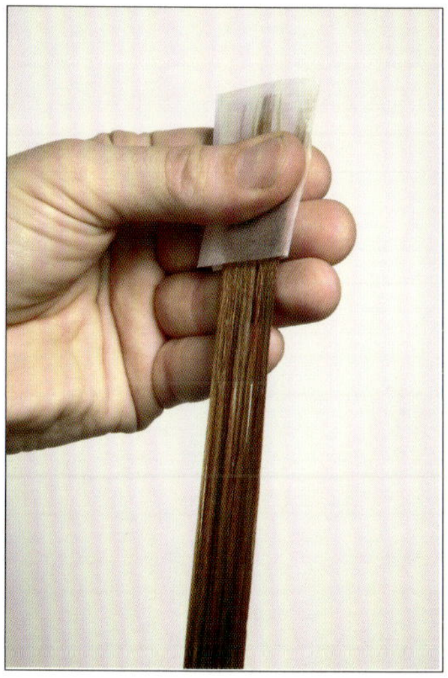
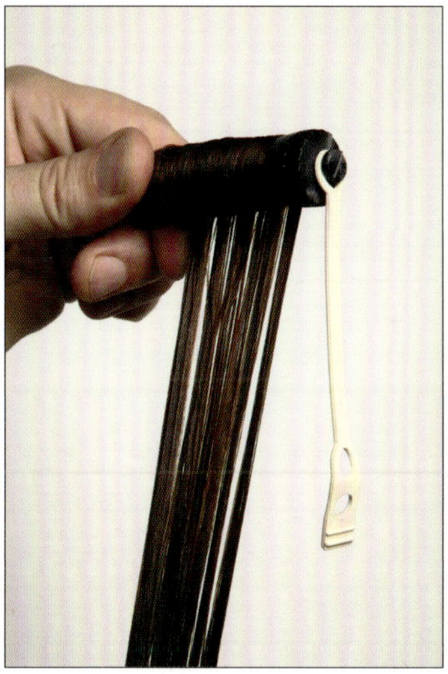
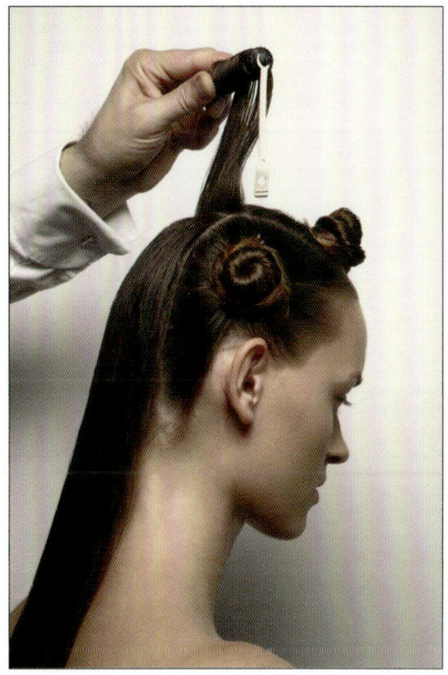
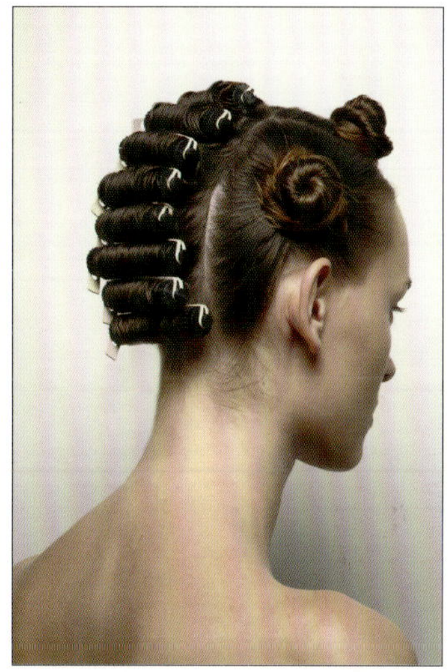

With a pin tail comb, take your first section horizontally just underneath the crown. Again the depth of your section should be about the same as the circumference of rod being used. Elevate this section up to 90 degrees, wrap an end paper around the ends of the hair and feed the section onto the rod, using the index finger and thumb of both hands. Wind the rod down to the roots and secure the rod with the rubber fastener, taking care not to position the rubber too close to the root area, as this may result in breaking the hair or leaving marks on the hair shaft after the perming process.

Continue taking sections down the back of the head and finishing on the hairline at the nape. Remember, while travelling down the back of the head, that the angle of your sections should follow the head's natural curvature when you elevate each subsequent section. The first panel of rods will now be in place.

Side Back Panel

From the radial section, wind the side back panel by taking horizontal sections across the head. Continue winding the rods behind the back of the ear and down towards the hairline in the nape area: remember to elevate each section by following the curvature of the head. It's important to maintain even tension while winding each section, and there should be no gaps between each panel of rods. This panel will now be complete. Repeat this process on the other side back panel of the head.

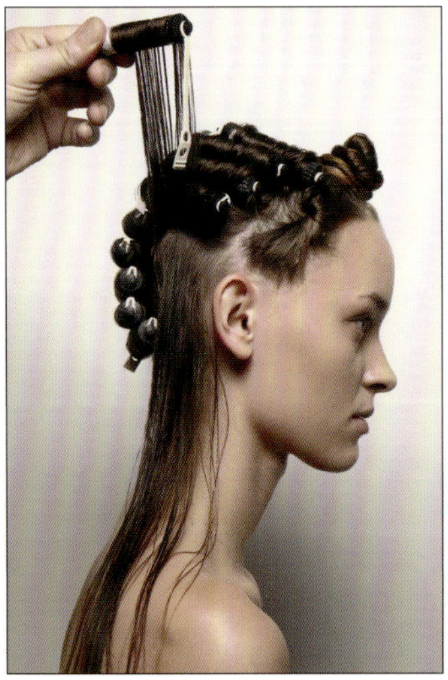 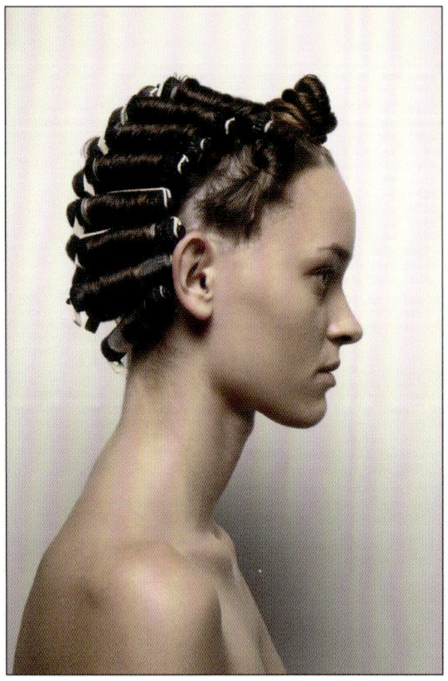 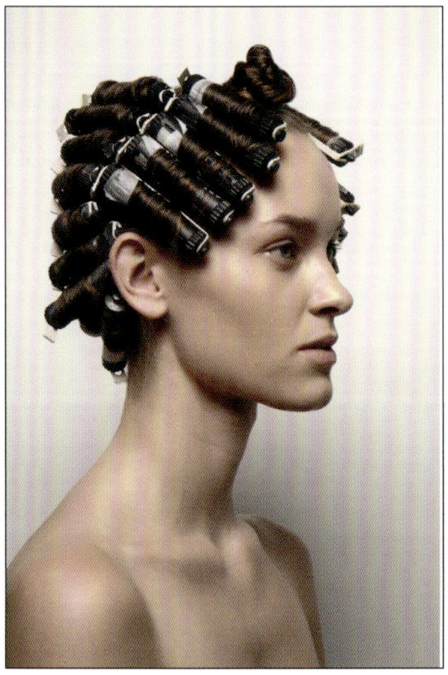 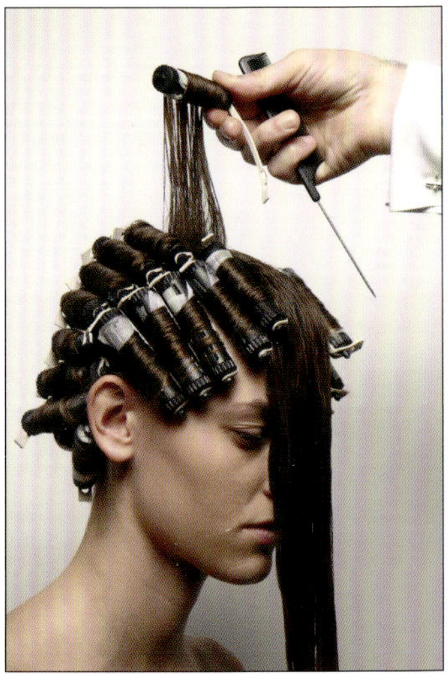

Side Front Panel

For the side front panel, take a horizontal section across this panel from the recession area on the front hairline. Elevate it and wind the rod, fasten in place, and continue working down towards the top of the ear, incorporating the hairline around the ear. This panel will now be complete.

Repeat this process on the other side of the head, starting at the side back panel and finishing on the side front panel. The winding of the perm will now be complete.

Be aware of keeping your sections all equally moist (slightly damp) during the winding process, as this will ensure even tension throughout and will not dilute the perm solution when you apply it.

Top Panel

Position yourself in front of your client: take a horizontal section from the crown and in front of the first rod you applied, and again elevate this section up to 90 degrees. Wrap an end paper around the ends of the hair and feed the section onto the rod by using the index finger and thumb of both hands. Wind the rod down to the roots and secure the rod with the rubber fastener. Continue winding this section to the front hairline. This panel will now be complete.

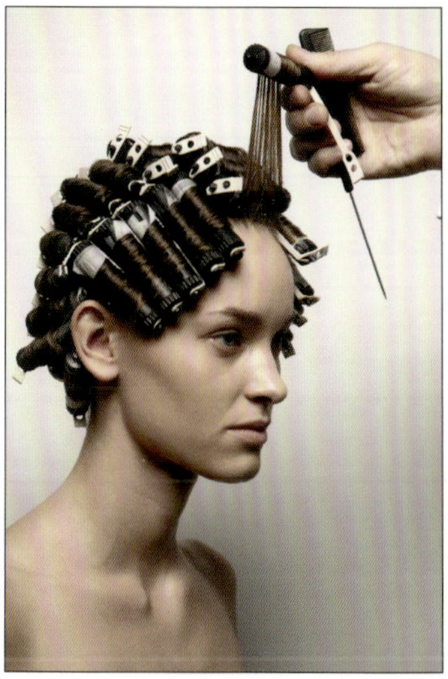

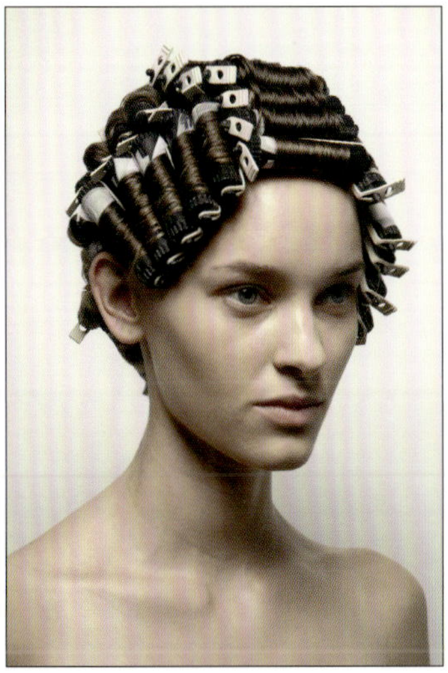

Barrier Cream

Distribute evenly a small amount of barrier cream around the client's entire hairline. This will help protect the skin from the chemicals in the perm solution. Next place a strip of cotton wool around the hairline – this will be held in place by the barrier cream by sticking to it. The cotton wool strip will protect the client and will help prevent any perm solution running off the rods onto the skin. Distribute the perm solution evenly over the rods. Excess perm solution may be absorbed by the cotton wool. When this happens, the cotton wool should be replaced to prevent the skin from being burnt.

Processing

Place a processing cap over the rods and fasten securely. Most perms are processed with heat from an accelerator, but make sure you follow the manufacturer's instructions. Check the processing at regular intervals. If you are using heat, allow the perm to cool and take a test curl: look for a good, even 'S' shape movement in the hair. The processing time will vary. The main factors are: room temperature, strength and pH of the perm solution, and the porosity and condition of the hair.

Once you have achieved the desired result, the perm is ready to be neutralised. For the neutralising process follow the manufacturer's instructions.

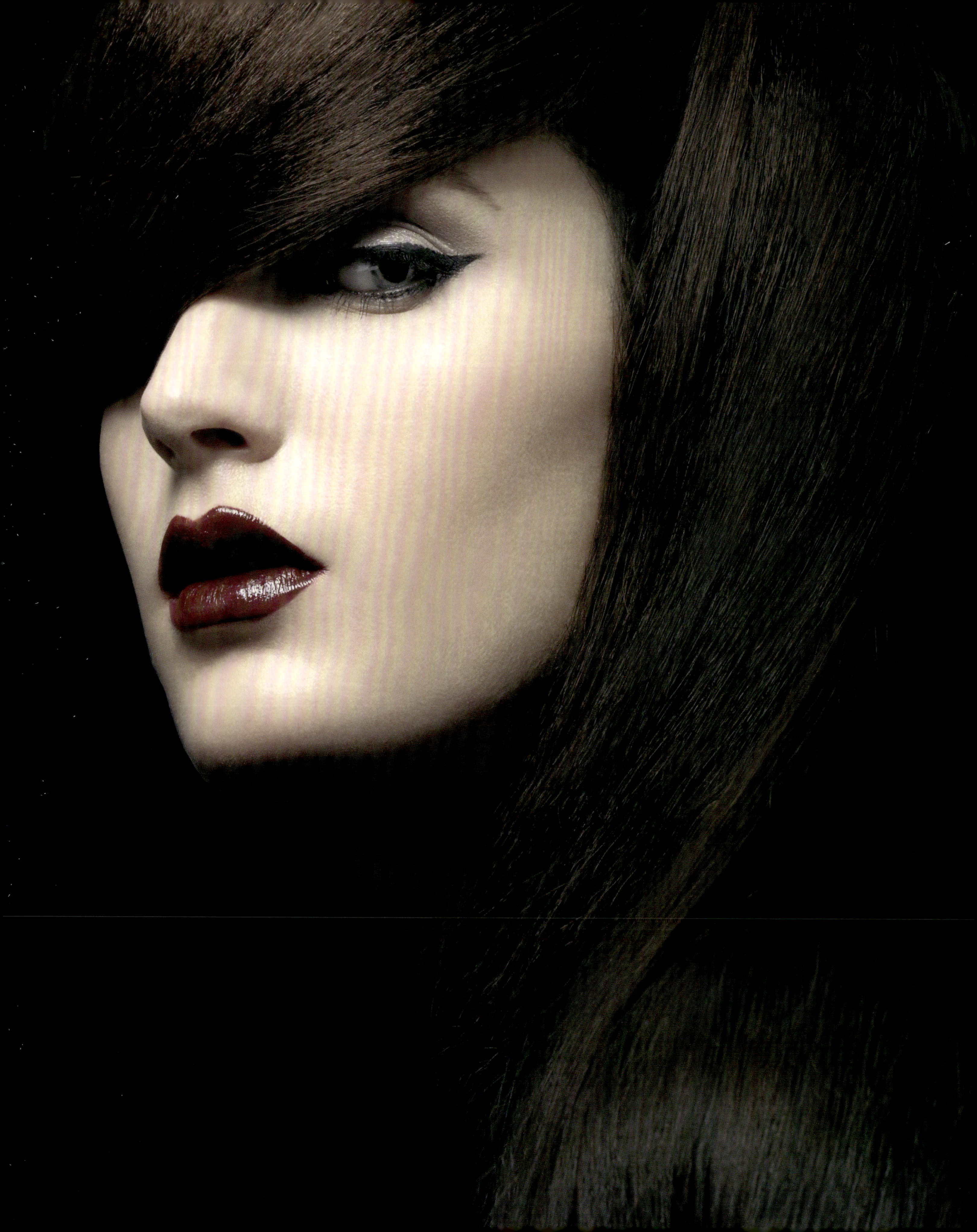

Interpreting Technique

At this stage of your journey you should be ready to look at interpreting the methods in *Technique*. As you develop your craft, take an idea and push it further. Experiment with hair, mix ideas and expand; play with colour, shape, texture and proportion.

The philosophy that creativity evolves from technique has developed from the belief that we learn to master skills in hairdressing, and these new found skills will give you the ability to create in an imaginative and inventive way. The tools that you'll need in order to carve a successful career in hairdressing can be found in the pages of this book. *Technique* provides a highly detailed approach that demonstrates disciplined ideas that will equip you with the essential knowledge that can help develop your own technique.

Recognising modern hairdressing as a mainstream consumer trend, men and women of all ages are investing time and money in the way their hair looks. The higher the quality of hairdressers' training, the more they can offer their clients.

By building on your skills, your interpretation and your signature will emerge. Try to be very open-minded to new ideas. It's all about technique in the first instance, and then how you use it.

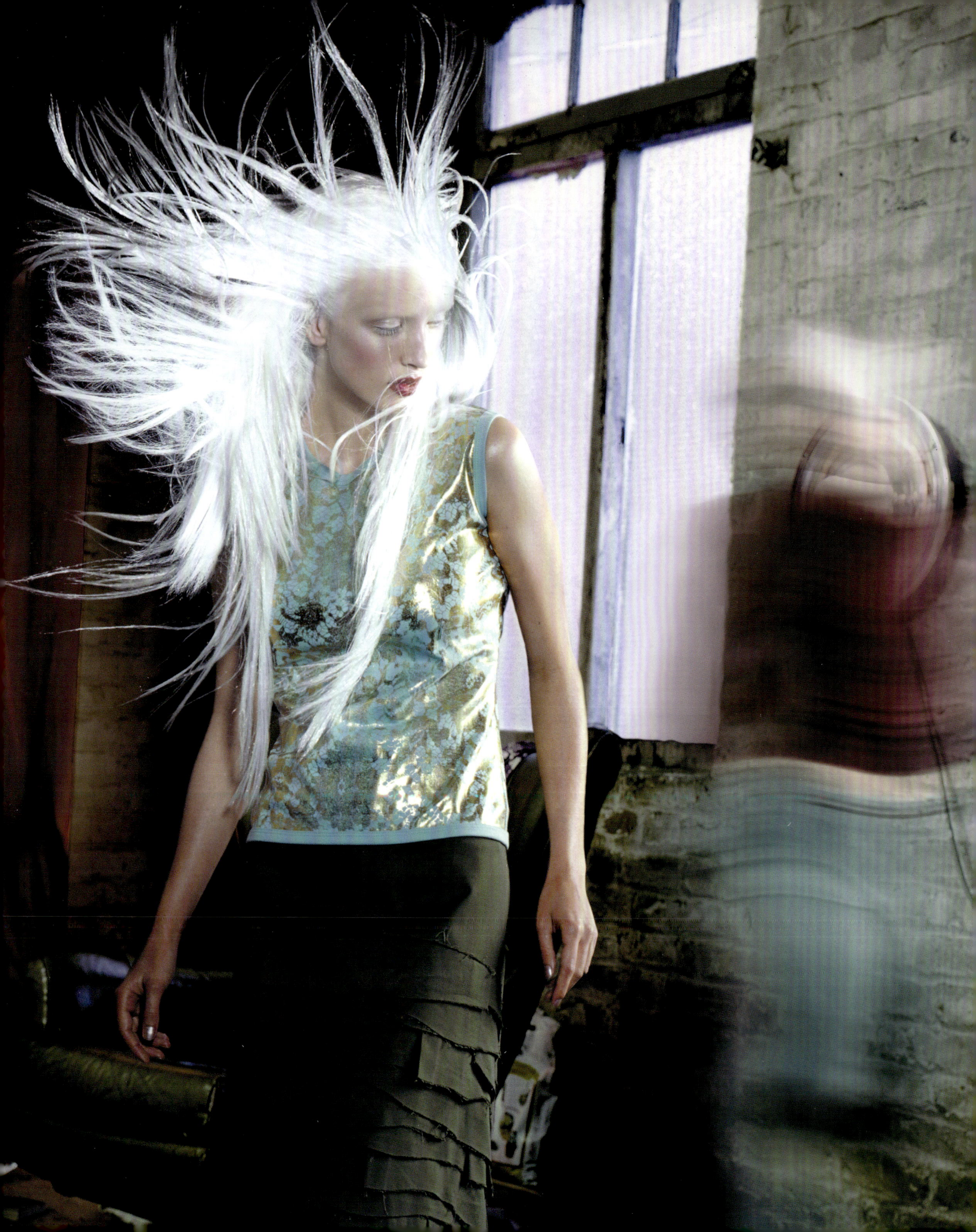

Session

The term 'session' in hairdressing usually refers to a hairdresser producing a hairstyle for a show, photograph, video or film. Session hairstylists would usually begin their careers by working with photographers, building their portfolio and testing with other creative people, such as make-up artists and fashion stylists. A test would bring together the team to develop and work on an idea for a photographic shoot. Ideally develop your book with a selection of images, best reflecting your signature look. A good way to start in session is to assist other session hairstylists at the shows, which are held bi-annually, or editorial/fashion/beauty shoots.

Try approaching an agency, as they may be able to put you in touch with someone who you could assist, it is also helpful to be represented by an agency specialising in this field. By having an agent, assignments will be much easier to secure, rather than by you approaching clients yourself. Some agencies deal with mainly commercial work aimed at the mass market. You may find yourself working on a shoot for a daily newspaper or weekly magazine. Other agencies are more exclusive and aim at the creative and luxury end of the market, working with high profile clients and prestigious accounts.

Very often session hairdressers are engaged in the fashion arena and will spend much of their time working on fashion shoots and catwalk shows. Music promos and film are other areas that one could be involved with. In the fashion world the seasons, spring/summer autumn/winter, play an important part especially if you are working on catwalk shows or fashion magazines. Fashion designers usually work six months to a year ahead. So the session hairdresser will need to complement the new seasonal trends by adapting and developing looks in hair alongside these trends. The trick is to keep a finger on the fashion pulse and be aware of new trends, especially in fashion and related areas.

Fashion

Fashion plays an integral part in the hairdressing industry. They work very closely together. Elements in fashion enable us to say something about ourselves and to the world around us. More importantly we express who we are or who we would like to be. The clothes and hairstyles we wear say a lot about us. They are our means of expression and communication to others. They reflect our need to belong to groups of people who dress in a similar way to ourselves, or share our lifestyle, profession or attitudes.

Fashion may also be used as a kind of protection or an armour. We could have a favourite piece of clothing which is special to us, something that flatters the body and boosts confidence, making us feel powerful, sexy, masculine or feminine. Trends come and go and fashion changes with the seasons. It's a process that has evolved over many years. As our culture and attitudes change, fashion changes along with it.

Hairdressing lends itself to fashion very willingly. They compliment each other perfectly, and there is a strong interest in total look, especially at the international catwalk shows and in photographic work. Hairdressers become fashionistas in their own right when working alongside other fashion industry professionals. We interpret ideas about hair into something real. The importance of fashion to the hairdresser is paramount. A strong interest in fashion, art, music, design and culture will prepare you for a highly rewarding career within the most exciting industry.

Hairdressing, fundamentally, is arranging a person's hair, be it for practical, decorative, ceremonial or symbolic reasons. From ancient times primitive men and women would plaster their hair with mud. Since then hair has been dyed, bleached, curled, texturised, braided, waxed, oiled, hennaed, powered, cut, shaved, enhanced with false hair, covered with wigs, hidden with nets, veils and all manner of headwear, and adorned with beads, jewels, combs, feathers, ribbons and flowers and other decorative elements.

In the world of fashion, hairdressing has always adapted and developed alongside it, and hairstyles, especially for women, have changed dramatically over the years. Hairstyles have been created and re-created – long to short and everything in between.

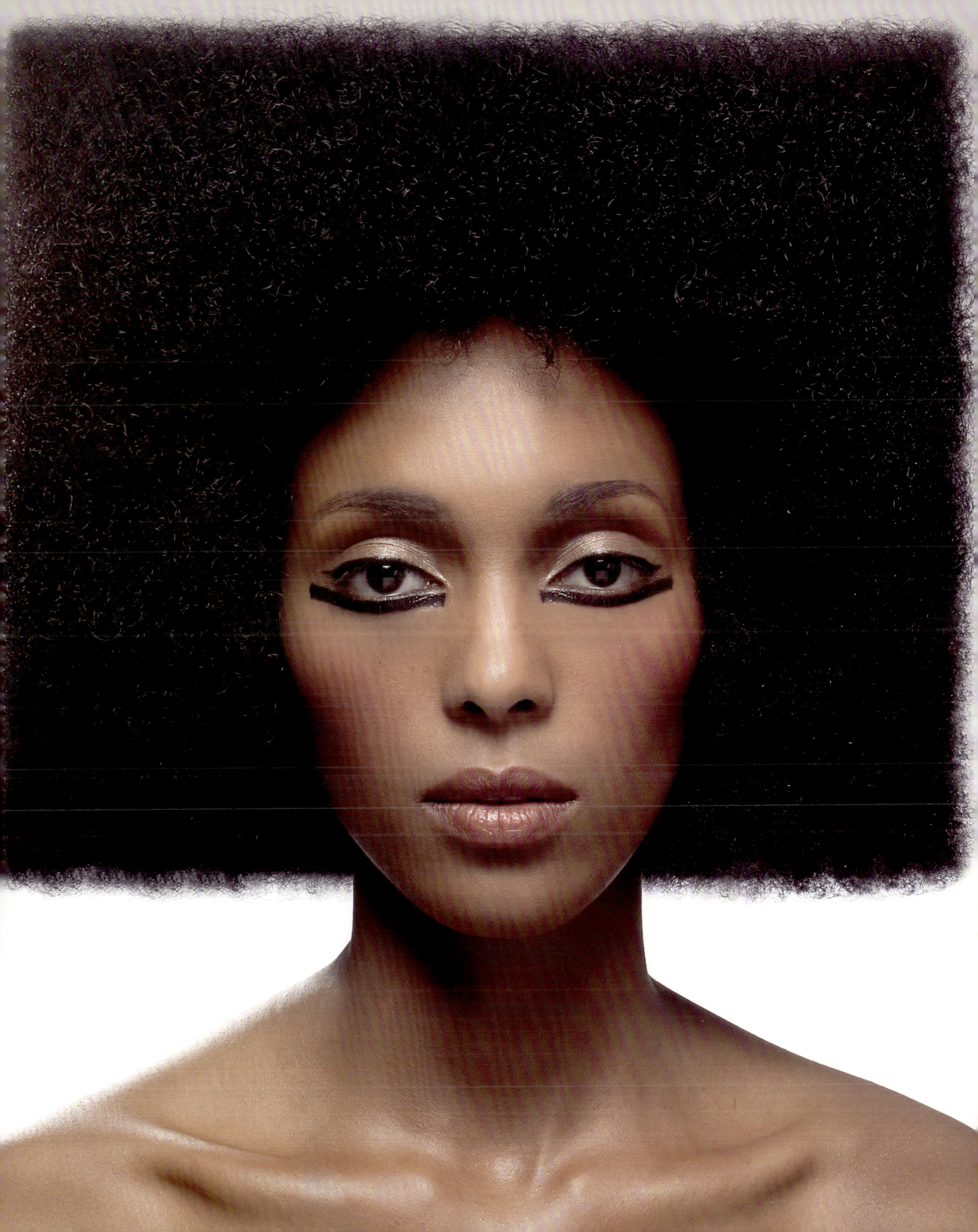

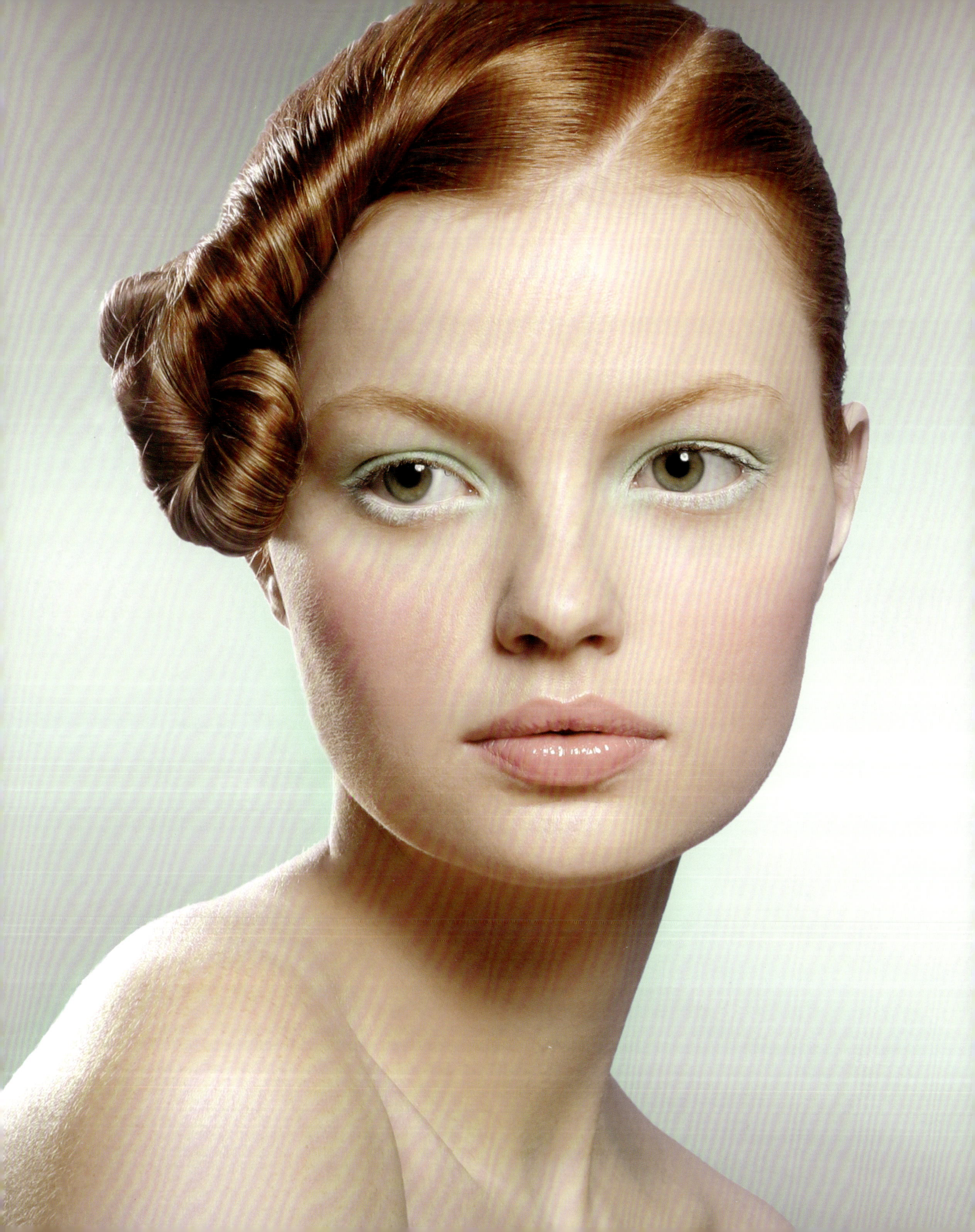

Hair Up

Dressing hair up works best on a length, on or below shoulder. Easy hair up styles range from simple ponytails and chignons to plaits and pleats. There are many variations of hair up styles to create, the following describes four basic hair up's.

Ponytails are simple to achieve when it comes to hair up. A very popular hairstyle that remains truly varied and versatile, generally the ponytail can be worn high on the head at the crown, or on the occipital bone, or at the base of the neck. A ponytail can be straightened or left in a natural wave, for more volume it can be curled and texturised.

Chignons are very easy hairstyles to create, a chignon can be made to look very clean or disheveled and can be placed at almost any position on the head. Hair pieces can be added to increase the size and texture of the chignon, the finish and texture will depend on the suitability and the occasion.

Pleats or vertical/horizontal rolls are usually worn at the back of the head. To begin, the hair is usually either wet or dry set in order to bulk up the hair and increase volume. To give a pleat support, volume and control, hair is back-combed. Pleats are held in place with grips and pins, which should not be seen in the finished result.

Plaits and braids are formed by intertwining sections of hair. Many intricate effects can be achieved, plaits can be worked on or off scalp. The most popular technique used for plaiting is a three section plait although plaits can be worked with many more sections to give an interesting, almost basket-like weave. Plaiting can be done on both wet or dry hair and on all hair types.

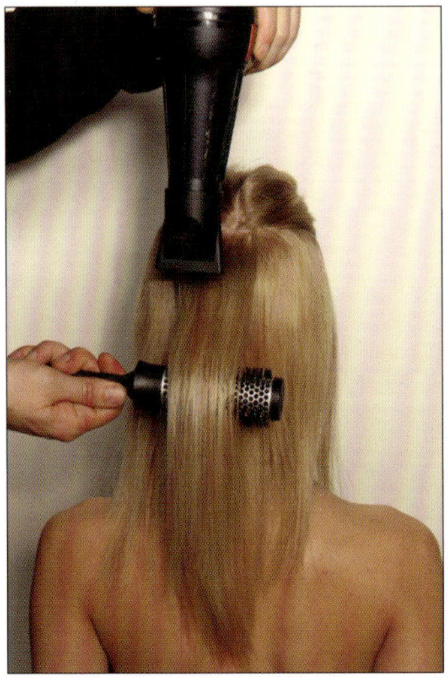
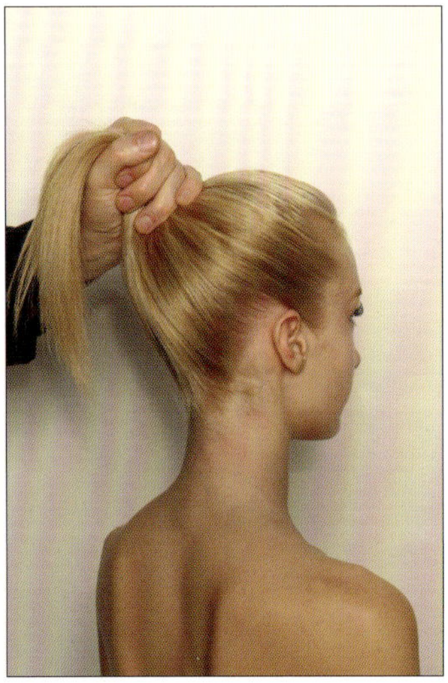
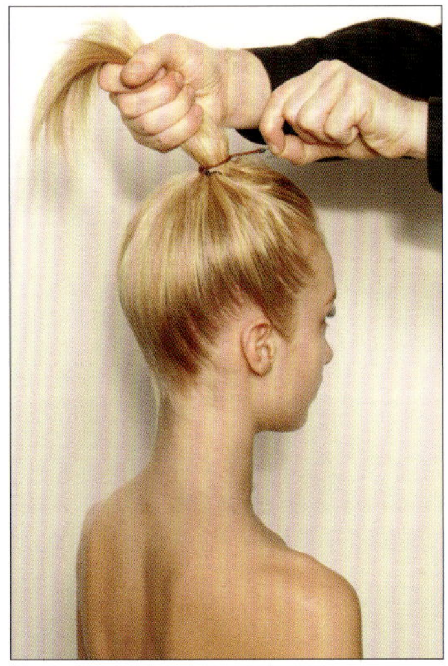
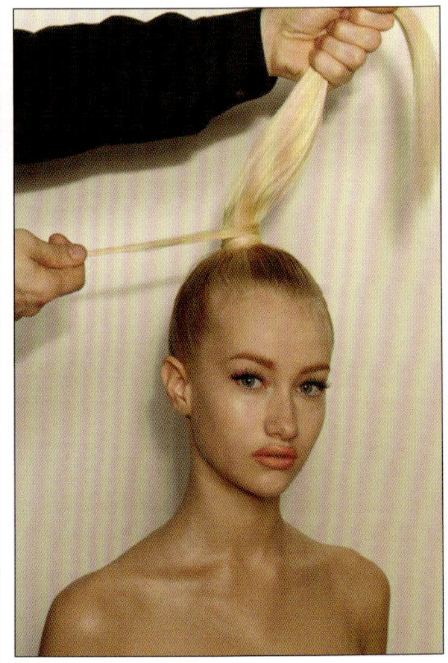

Ponytail

1 Prepare the hair by smoothing out the surface by means of blow drying, use the correct styling product to give hold, control, volume and shine as necessary. Pay particular attention around the hairline when smoothing out. Once the hair has been prepared a finishing product may be applied and distributed throughout the hair, this also depends on the required result.

2 Decide where on the head to position the ponytail. Brush through the hair and up from the entire hairline and start to gather the hair into the palm of the hand.

3 Grasp the base of the ponytail between the thumb and index finger, hook on a bungee at the base of the ponytail, wrap it around the base securely and fix the hook in place. Bungees are made from elastic with a metallic hook on each end, they are approximately 10cms long and available in packs. They are also available in black, brown or beige. Always match the colour of the bungee to your clients hair.

4 To hide the bungee used to hold the ponytail in place, take a section of hair from underneath the ponytail, wrap it around the base of the ponytail to cover the elastic, secure underneath with a pin. Dress or texturise as required.

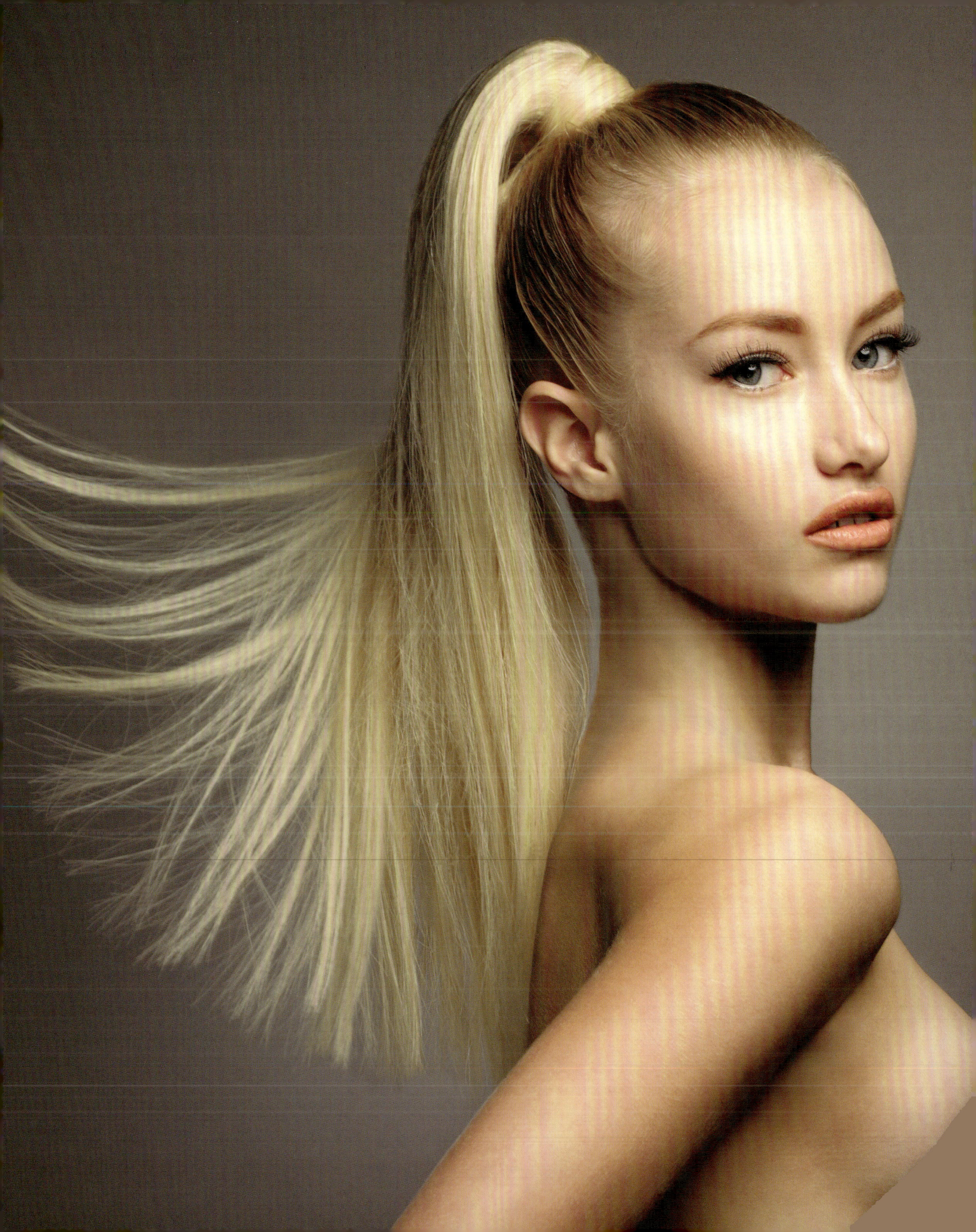

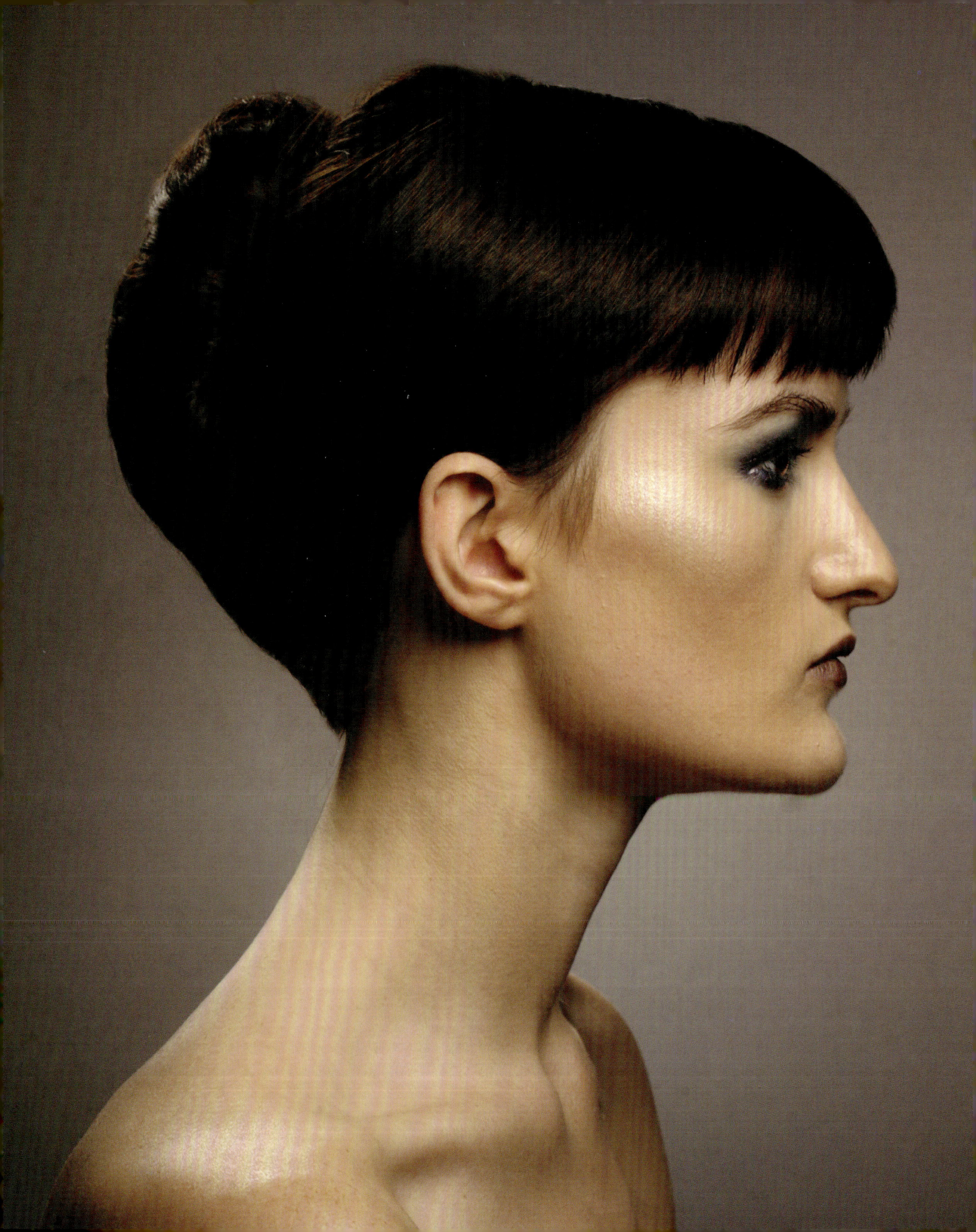

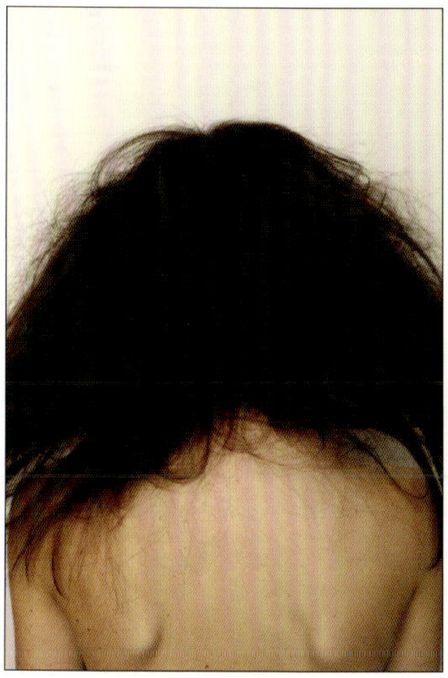

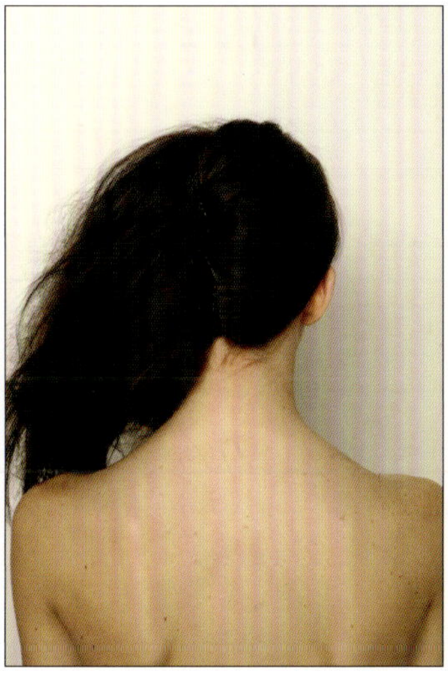

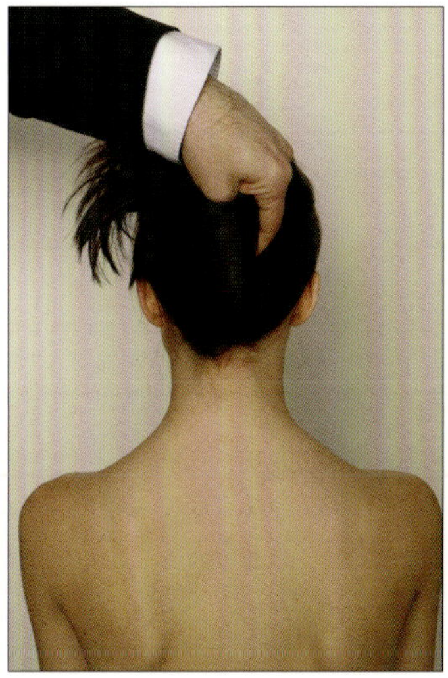

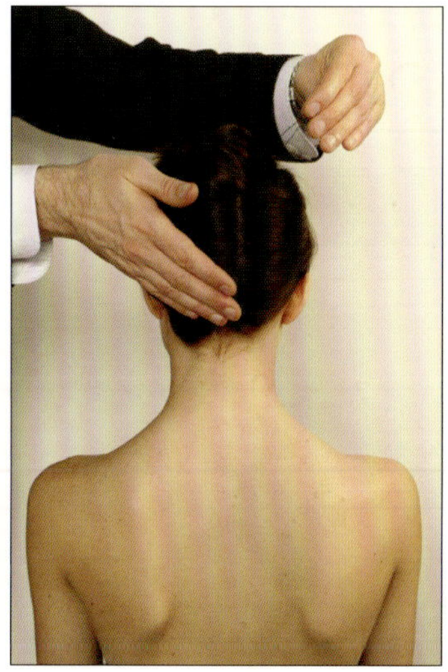

Pleat

1 Prepare by deciding on the required finish of the hair, for example, blow dry for a smooth and glossy finish, setting bulks up the hair, for a dense matte finish ruffle the surface of each section between the palms of the hands, use appropriate styling products. Progress by back combing all the hair. To back-comb, take a section of hair and hold it firmly between the thumb and index finger of one hand, with a comb or brush push down about an inch away from the roots and continue along to the mid-lengths and ends. Back-combing underneath the section gives bulk, back-combing on top of the section gives control. Smooth over the top of the back-combed section to give a neat finish. Work in vertical sections from below a horse-shoe section, work evenly and technically. Create a uniform back-combed texture throughout.

2 Using a natural bristle brush, work from the front hairline incorporating the temple area and around the ear and brush back horizontally. Use as much or as little tension as required. Start working off centre and from the hairline at the nape, criss-cross a line of hair grips, finishing just below the crown.

3 From the front hair line on the other side of the head, brush back the entire section horizontally. Gather the section into the palm of the hand and twist around the thumb, the ends are tucked inside and the pleat is formed, secure the pleat with hair pins making sure they are not visible. At this stage, the sections worked so far incorporated into the pleat should be horizontal.

4 Work the top and front section back away from the front hair line and tuck the ends underneath the pleat at the crown area. Remember to check balance. There are many variations on the pleat, the example shown incorporates a parting and a fringe. Extra height may be required through the top, its a question of suitability.

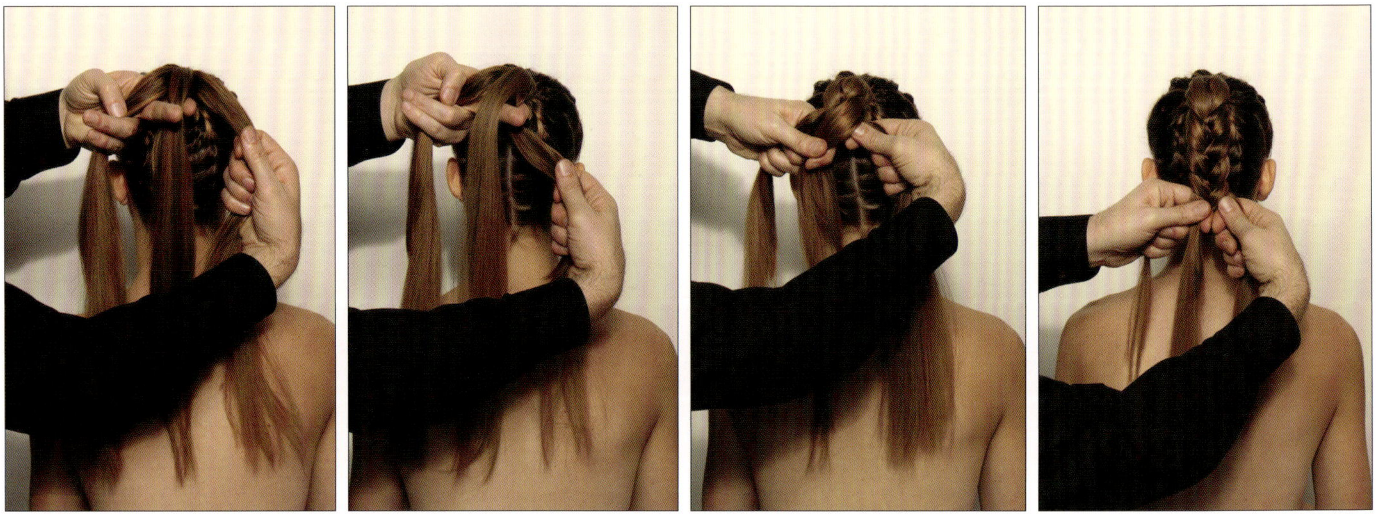

Plait

1 Prepare the hair as to the desired finish, if necessary using styling products as required. Decide where to position the plait (in this instance working off scalp at the crown). Form a pony-tail and divide the hair into three equal sections.

2 Take the section on the right side and cross it over the middle section, maintain a certain degree of even tension throughout when working the sections. Hold the sections firmly between the index finger and thumb of each hand.

3 Take the left section and cross it over the section which is now in the middle, again keeping a good tension throughout the progression.

4 Repeat and take the right section and cross it over the middle section. Continue until reaching the end of the length of the plait being worked. Sections on either side cross over the middle section and in turn become the middle section. The middle section is never handled. Only the left and right sections are crossed over the middle to become the middle section in their turn. Secure the end of the plait with covered elastic.

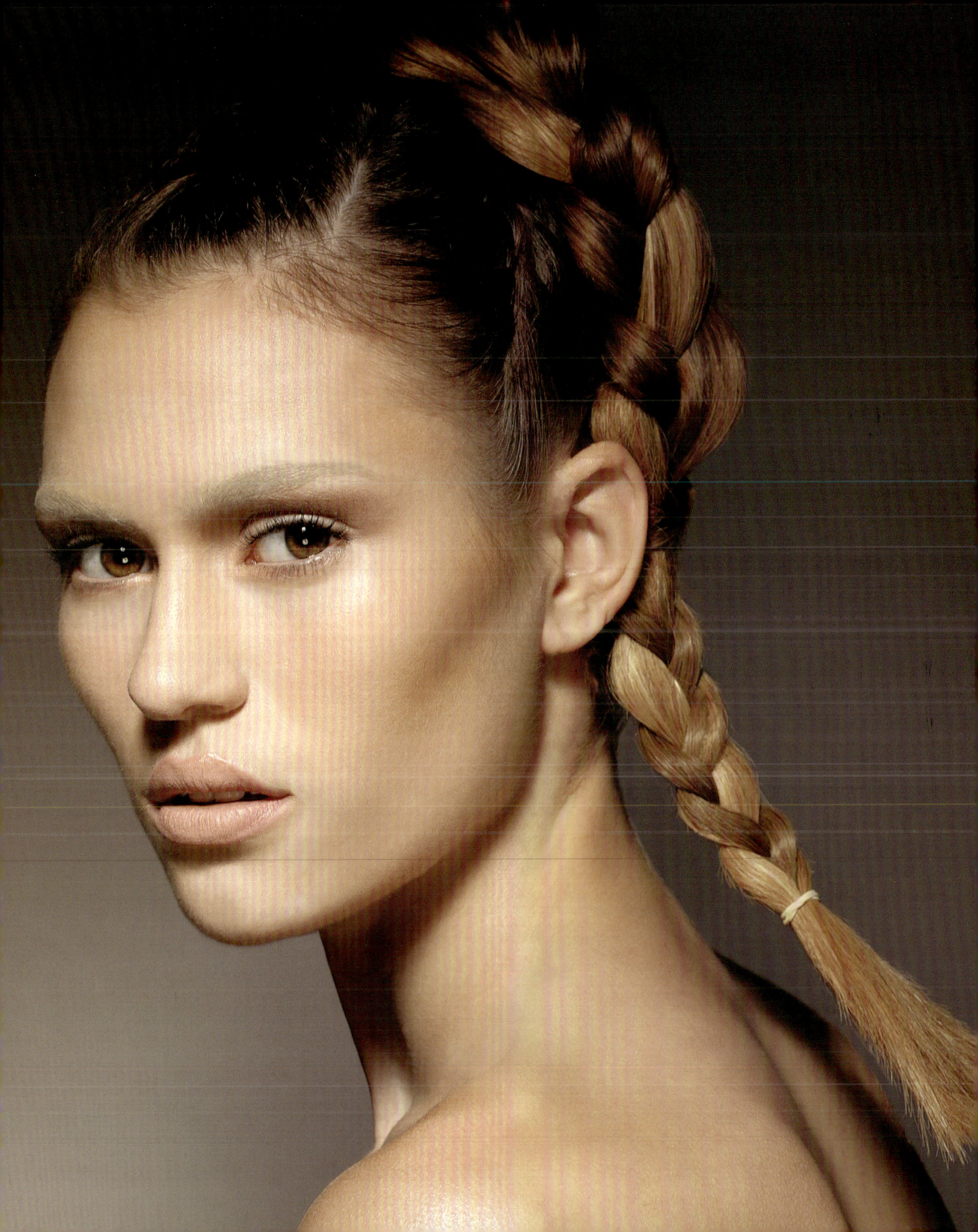

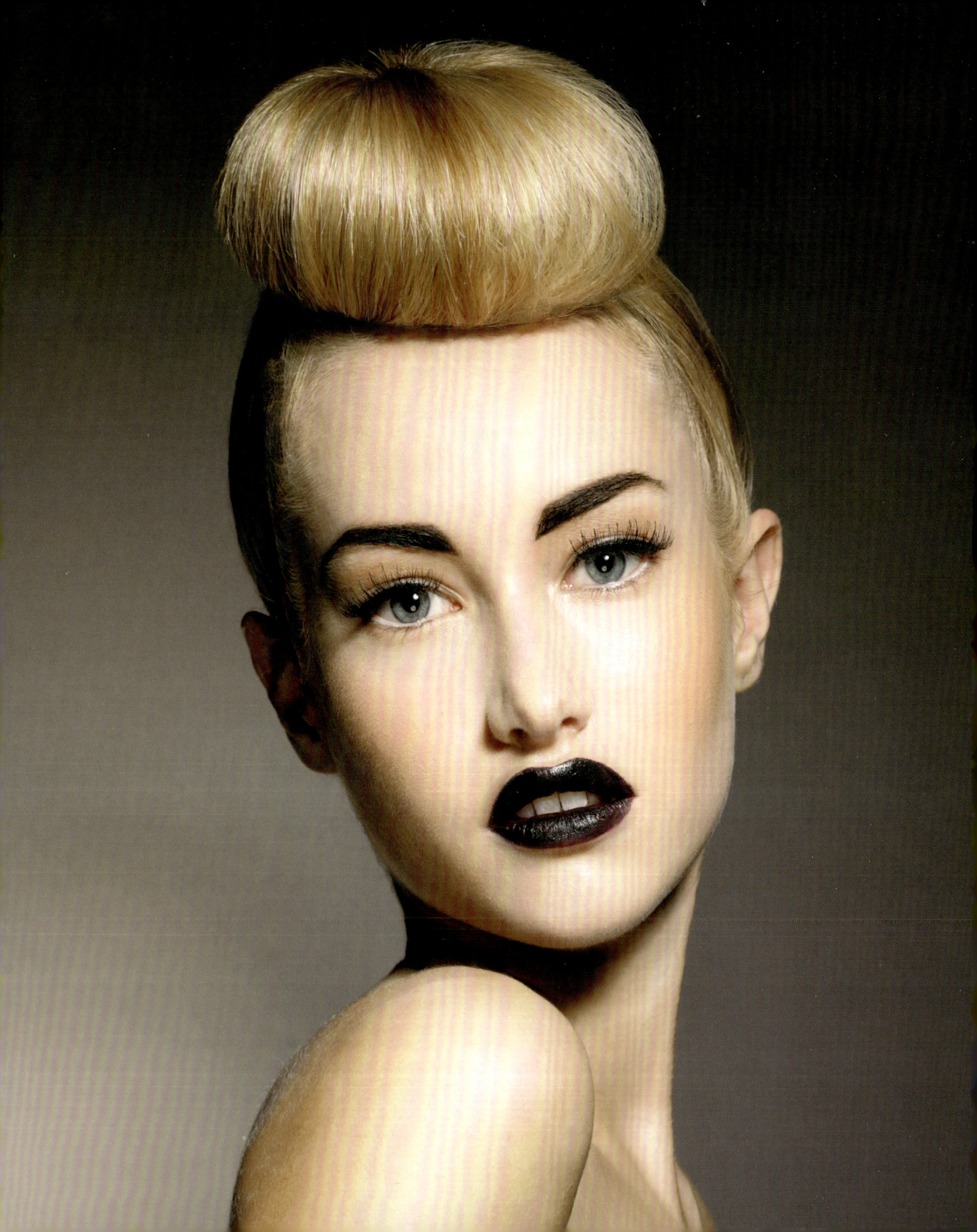

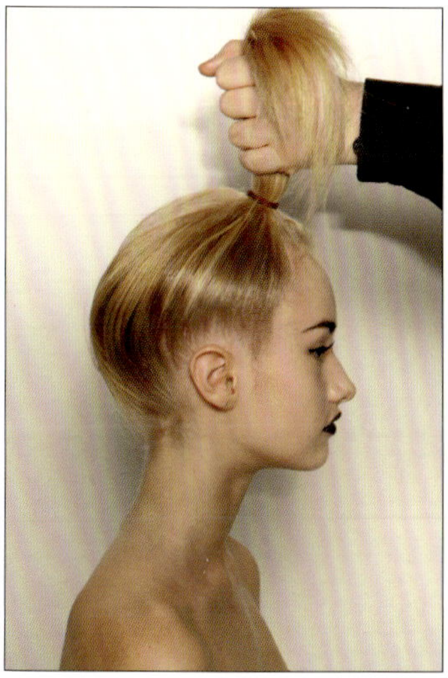
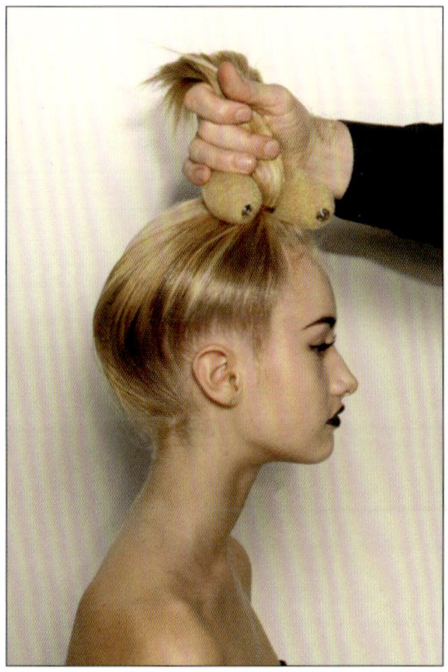
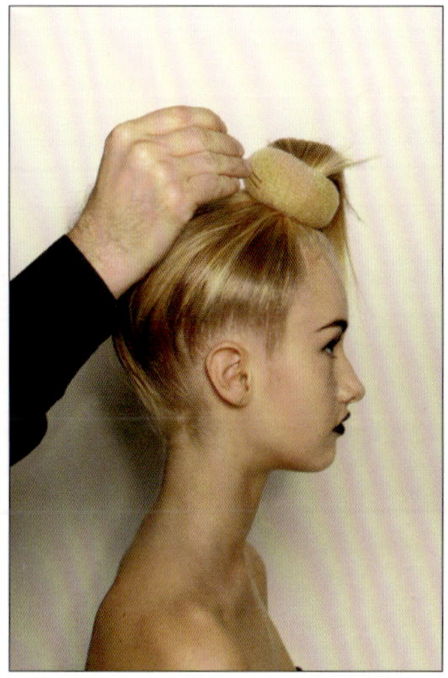
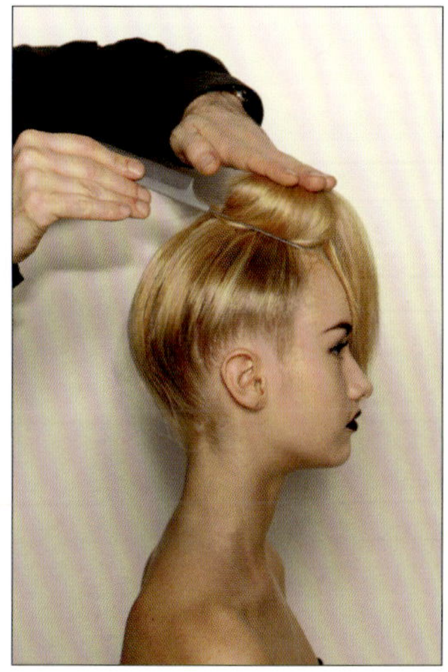

Chignon

1 Prepare the hair by smoothing out the surface by means of blow drying or setting, setting the hair will give a bend to the hair making it slightly easier to work with, this will add bulk and volume. Use the appropriate styling product to give hold, control, volume and shine as necessary. Once the hair has been prepared a finishing product may be applied and distributed throughout the hair, this also depends on the required result. Pay particular attention around the hairline when smoothing out.

2 Decide where on the head to position the chignon and brush through and up from the entire hairline and start to gather the hair into the palm of the hand and secure with a bungee at the base.

3 Wrap a padded support around the base and fix in place securely with hair pins, divide the hair equally and dress the hair over the support using a pintail comb to tuck the ends underneath the support. Finally, pin in place making sure that the pins are not visible.

4 Alternatively, if a support is not required, twist the entire length of the section all the way to the end, wrap the twisted section back on itself around the base tucking the ends underneath the chignon, secure with hair pins.

Index

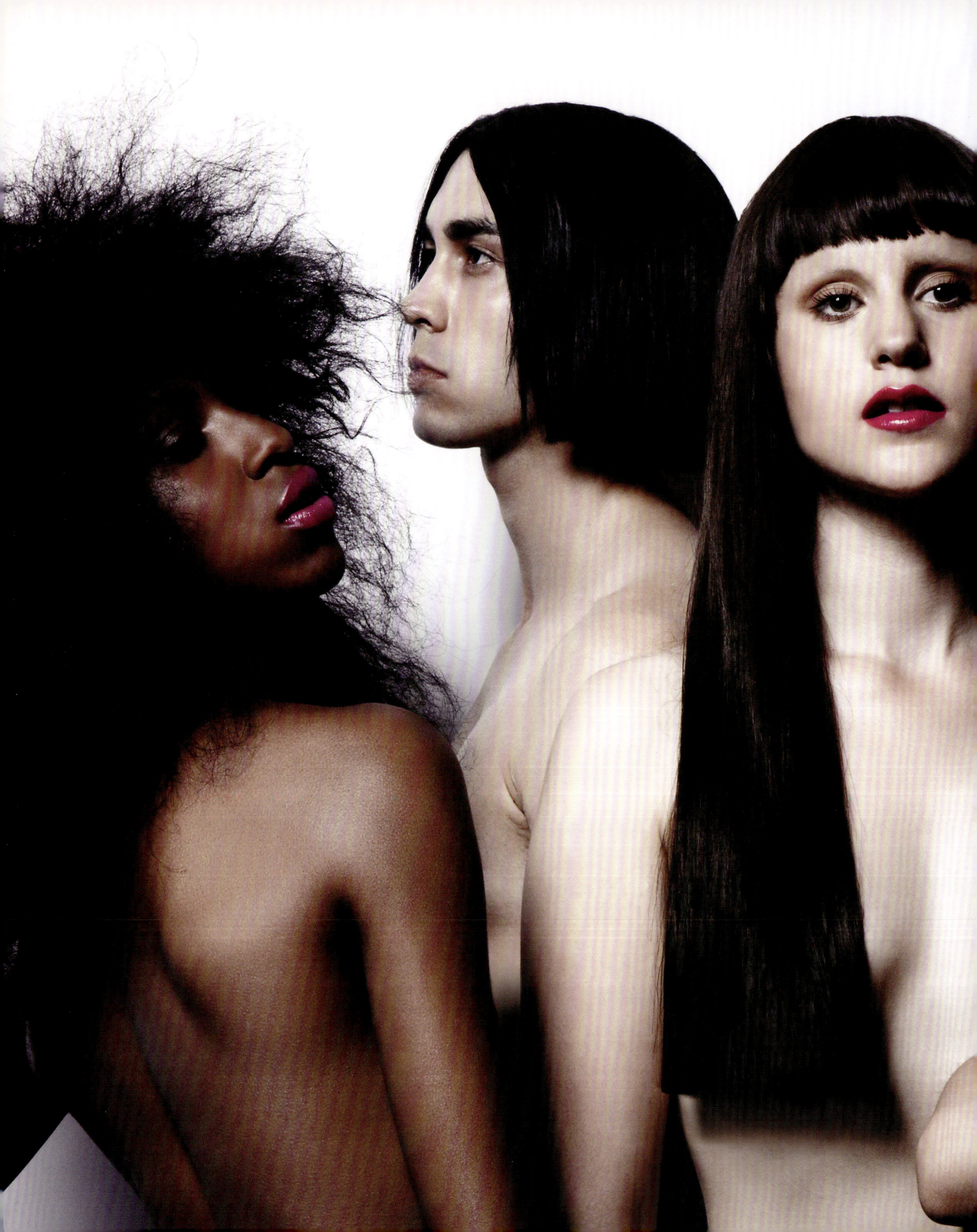

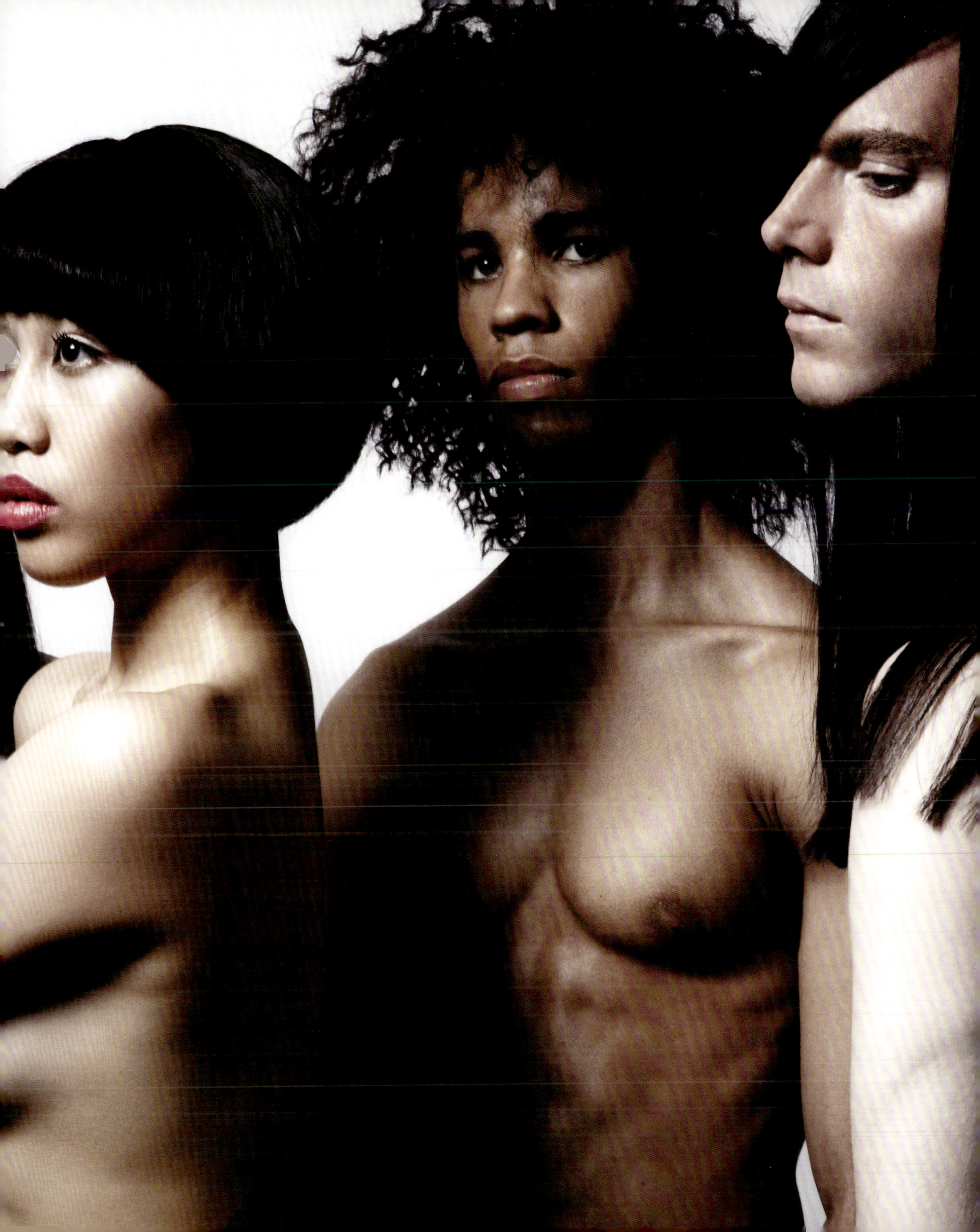

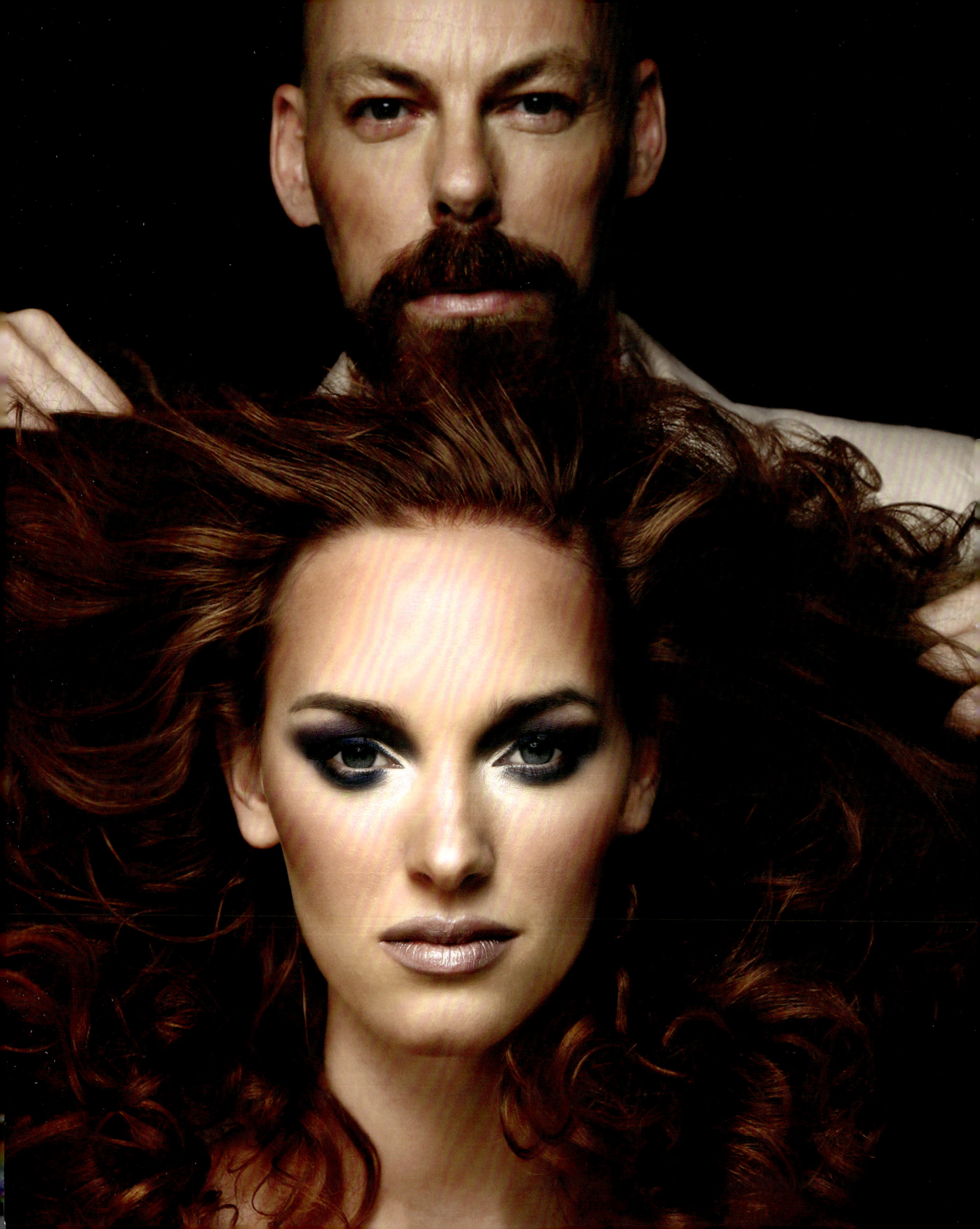